Contents

How This Book Can Help You Learn iv

Note-Taking Tips v

Chapter 1: Community Health: Yesterday, Today, and Tomorrow 1

Chapter 2: Organizations That Help Shape Community Health 11

Chapter 3: Epidemiology: The Study of Disease, Injury, and Death in the Community 21

Chapter 4: Epidemiology: Prevention and Control of Diseases and Health Conditions 31

Chapter 5: Community Organizing/Building and Health Promotion Programming 41

Chapter 6: The School Health Program: A Component of Community Health 51

Chapter 7: Maternal, Infant, and Child Health 57

Chapter 8: Adolescents, Young Adults, and Adults 73

Chapter 9: Elders 81

Chapter 10: Community Health and Minorities 93

Chapter 11: Community Mental Health 107

Chapter 12: Alcohol, Tobacco, and Other Drugs: A Community Concern 117

Chapter 13: Health Care System: Structure 129

Chapter 14: Health Care System: Function 141

Chapter 15: Environmental Concerns: Wastes and Pollution 155

Chapter 16: The Impact of Environment on Human Health 167

Chapter 17: Injuries as a Community Health Problem 177

Chapter 18: Safety and Health in the Workplace 191

How This Book Can Help You Learn

All of us have different learning styles. Some of us are visual learners, some more auditory, some learn better by doing an activity. Some students prefer to learn new material using visual aids. Some learn material better when they hear it in a lecture; others learn it better by reading it. Cognitive research has shown that no matter what your learning style, you will learn more if you are actively engaged in the learning process.

This Student Note-Taking Guide will help you learn by providing a structure to your notes and letting you utilize all of the learning styles mentioned above. Students don't need to copy down every word their professor says or recopy their entire textbook. Do the assigned reading, listen in lecture, follow the key points your instructor is making, and write down meaningful notes. After reading and lectures, review your notes and pull out the most important points.

The Student Note-Taking Guide is your partner and guide in note-taking. Your Guide provides you with a visual guide that follows the chapter topics presented in your textbook. If your instructor is using the PowerPoint slides that accompany the text, this guide will save you from having to write down everything that is on the slides. There is space provided for you to jot down the terms and concepts that you feel are most important to each lecture. By working with your Guide, you are seeing, hearing, writing, and, later, reading and reviewing. The more often you are exposed to the material, the better you will learn and understand it. Using different methods of exposure significantly increases your comprehension.

Your Guide is the perfect place to write down questions that you want to ask your professor later, interesting ideas that you want to discuss with your study group, or reminders to yourself to go back and study a certain concept again to make sure that you really got it.

Having organized notes is essential at exam time and when doing homework assignments. Your ability to easily locate the important concepts of a recent lecture will help you move along more rapidly, as you don't have to spend time rereading an entire chapter just to reinforce one point that you may not have quite understood.

Your Guide is a valuable resource. You've found a wonderful study partner!

Note-Taking Tips

1. It is easier to take notes if you are not hearing the information for the first time. Read the chapter or the material that is about to be discussed before class. This will help you to anticipate what will be said in class, and have an idea of what to write down. It will also help to read over your notes from the last class. This way you can avoid having to spend the first few minutes of class trying to remember where you left off last time.

2. Don't waste your time trying to write down everything that your professor says. Instead, listen closely and only write down the important points. Review these important points after class to help remind you of related points that were made during the lecture.

3. If the class discussion takes a spontaneous turn, pay attention and participate in the discussion. Only take notes on the conclusions that are relevant to the lecture.

4. Emphasize main points in your notes. You may want to use a highlighter, special notation (asterisks, exclamation points), format (circle, underline), or placement on the page (indented, bulleted). You will find that when you try to recall these points, you will be able to actually picture them on the page.

5. Be sure to copy down word-for-word specific formulas, laws, and theories.

6. Hearing something repeated, stressed, or summed up can be a signal that it is an important concept to understand.

7. Organize handouts, study guides, and exams in your notebook along with your lecture notes. It may be helpful to use a three-ring binder, so that you can insert pages wherever you need to.

8. When taking notes, you might find it helpful to leave a wide margin on all four sides of the page. Doing this allows you to note names, dates, definitions, etc., for easy access and studying later. It may also be helpful to make notes of questions you want to ask your professor about or research later, ideas or relationships that you want to explore more on your own, or concepts that you don't fully understand.

9. It is best to maintain a separate notebook for each class. Labeling and dating your notes can be helpful when you need to look up information from previous lectures.

10. Make your notes legible, and take notes directly in your notebook. Chances are you won't recopy them no matter how noble your intentions. Spend the time you would have spent recopying the notes studying them instead, drawing conclusions and making connections that you didn't have time for in class.

11. Look over your notes after class while the lecture is still fresh in your mind. Fix illegible items and clarify anything you don't understand. Do this again right before the next class.

Notes

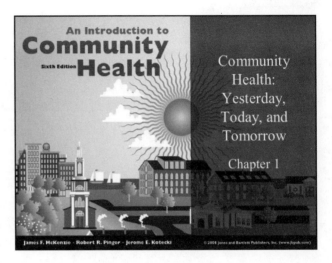

Introduction

- **Much progress was made in the 20th century**
- **Still room for improvement**
  - Health behavior
  - Noninfectious diseases, e.g., diabetes, heart disease
  - Infectious diseases e.g., pan flu, drug-resistant pathogens
  - Terrorism
- **Good health remains a goal worldwide**

© 2008 Jones and Bartlett Publishers, Inc. (www.jbpub.com)

Definitions - 1

- **Health**
  - "A state of complete physical, mental, and social well being and not merely the absence of disease and infirmity" (WHO, 1947)

  - A *dynamic* state or condition of the human organism that is multi-dimensional in nature, a resource for living, and results from a person's interactions with and adaptations to his or her environment

© 2008 Jones and Bartlett Publishers, Inc. (www.jbpub.com)

Notes

_____

Definitions - 2

- **Community**
  - Group of people who have common characteristics; can be defined by location, race, ethnicity, age, occupation, interest, or other common bond
  - Characteristics of communities:
    1. Membership
    2. Common symbol system
    3. Shared values and norms
    4. Mutual influence
    5. Shared needs and commitment
    6. Shared emotional connection

© 2008 Jones and Bartlett Publishers, Inc. (www.jbpub.com)

Definitions - 3

- **Public health** – "what we as a society do collectively to assure the conditions in which people can be healthy" (IOM, 1988)
- **Community health** – the health status of a defined group of people and the actions and conditions to promote, protect, and preserve their health
- **Population health** – the health status of people who are not organized and have no identity as a group or locality and the actions and conditions to promote, protect, and preserve their health

© 2008 Jones and Bartlett Publishers, Inc. (www.jbpub.com)

Community Health versus Personal Health

- **Community health activities**
  - Those aimed at protecting or improving the health of a population or community

- **Personal health activities**
  - Individual actions and decision-making that affect the health of an individual or his or her immediate family

© 2008 Jones and Bartlett Publishers, Inc. (www.jbpub.com)

Factors Affecting Community Health

- **Physical factors** – industrial development, community size, environment, geography
- **Social and cultural factors** – beliefs, traditions, prejudices, economics, politics, religion, socioeconomic status, social norms
- **Community organization** – identify problem, mobilize resources, work toward change
- **Individual behaviors** – takes the concerted effort of many—if not most—to improve community health

© 2008 Jones and Bartlett Publishers, Inc. (www.jbpub.com)

Brief History of Community and Public Health - 1

- **Earliest Civilizations**
  - Predate archaeological records
- **Ancient Societies (before *500 B.C.*)**
  - Northern India: evidence of bathrooms & sewers
  - Middle Kingdom of ancient Egypt: evidence of water drainage
  - Crete: evidence of toilets, flushing systems, & sewers
  - Sumerian clay tablet: Evidence of prescription drugs
  - Guides: Code of Hammurabi; Book of Leviticus

© 2008 Jones and Bartlett Publishers, Inc. (www.jbpub.com)

Brief History of Community and Public Health - 2

- **Classical Cultures *(500 B.C.–A.D. 500)***
  - Greeks: Used information from earlier groups; during "Golden age" men participated in games of strength & skill; active in community sanitation; running water; supplemented local city wells with water supplies from mountains as far as 10 miles away
  - Romans: Improved on Greek engineering & built aqueducts & sewer systems; Christians built hospitals for the public as charitable organizations

© 2008 Jones and Bartlett Publishers, Inc. (www.jbpub.com)

Brief History of Community and Public Health - 3

- **Middle Ages** *(A.D. 500–1500)*; **Dark Ages** *(A.D. 500–1000)*
  - Growing revulsion of the Roman materialism & spirituality
  - Spiritual era of public health
  - Great epidemics of plague
  - Recognizable diseases & many unidentifiable
  - Last epidemic of period–syphilis

© 2008 Jones and Bartlett Publishers, Inc. (www.jbpub.com)

Brief History of Community and Public Health - 4

- **Renaissance & Exploration** *(1500–1700)*
  - Rebirth of thinking about nature of the world and of humankind
  - More careful accounting of who was getting sick (saints and sinners both)
  - Belief that diseases were caused by environmental, not spiritual, factors
  - Observed the sick, leading to a greater understanding of signs and symptoms of a disease

© 2008 Jones and Bartlett Publishers, Inc. (www.jbpub.com)

Brief History of Community and Public Health - 5

- **The 18th Century**
  - Industrial growth
  - Cities overcrowded; water supplies inadequate; streets heaped with trash & garbage
  - Workplaces unsafe and unhealthy
  - 1790: First U.S. census
  - 1796: Dr. Jenner demonstrated smallpox vaccination
  - 1798: Marine Hospital Service (becomes U.S.P.H.S)
  - 1799: Large city boards of health

© 2008 Jones and Bartlett Publishers, Inc. (www.jbpub.com)

Brief History of
Community and Public Health - 6

- **The 19th Century (1st half)**
  - Few advancements in public health

  - Federal government approach *laissez faire*

  - Health quackery thrived

  - Epidemics continued: London cholera epidemics;
    Miasmas theory of contagious disease

Brief History of
Community and Public Health - 7

- **The 19th Century (2nd half)**
  - 1850: Modern era of public health begins
  - 1850: Shattuck's report
  - 1854: Snow removes pump handle
  - 1863: Pasteur proposed germ theory
  - 1872: APHA founded
  - 1876: Koch established relationship–microbe & disease
  - 1900: Reed announced yellow fever transmitted by
    mosquitoes

Brief History of
Community and Public Health - 8

- **Modern era of public health (1850 to present)**
  - Miasma, 1850 to 1875

  - Bacteriological, 1875 to 1900

  - Health Resources Development, 1900 to 1960

  - Social Engineering, 1960 to 1975

  - Health Promotion, 1975 to present

Notes

Notes

Brief History of Community and Public Health - 9

- **The 20th Century**
  - 1900-1920: Reform Phase
  - 1900: Life expectancy < 50 years
  - 1902: First voluntary health agency
  - 1906: Sinclair's *The Jungle* published
  - 1911: First local health department
  - 1918: Birth of school health
  - 1918: First school of public health in U.S.

© 2008 Jones and Bartlett Publishers, Inc. (www.jbpub.com)

Brief History of Community and Public Health - 10

- **The 20th Century (continued)**
  - 1922: Wood created first professional preparation for health educators
  - 1933: New Deal; unsuccessful attempt at national health care program
  - 1935: Social Security Act
  - 1946: Hill-Burton Act
  - 1952: Polio vaccine
  - 1965: Medicare & Medicaid bills passed
  - 1970: OSHA Act

© 2008 Jones and Bartlett Publishers, Inc. (www.jbpub.com)

Brief History of Community and Public Health - 11

- **Period of Health Promotion (1974-present)**
  - 1974: *A New Perspective on Health of Canadians* published
  - 1976: Health Information and Health Promotion Act passed
  - 1977: WHO's "Health for All"
  - 1979: *Healthy People* published
  - 1980: First set of national goals & objectives published
  - 1990: *Healthy People 2000* published
  - 2000: *Healthy People 2010* published

© 2008 Jones and Bartlett Publishers, Inc. (www.jbpub.com)

Community Health in the Early 2000s

- **Issues ahead**
  - Health care delivery
  - Environmental problems
  - Lifestyle diseases
  - Communicable diseases
  - Alcohol and other drug abuse
  - Disasters

© 2008 Jones and Bartlett Publishers, Inc. (www.jbpub.com)

Community Health in the Early 2000s - 2

- **Health Care Delivery**
  - Costs: 16% GDP, $2.2 trillion

  - Uninsured: 46.6 million

  - Access

  - National health insurance?

© 2008 Jones and Bartlett Publishers, Inc. (www.jbpub.com)

Community Health in the Early 2000s - 3

- **Environmental problems**
  - Pollution of water, air, & soil

  - Disposal of wastes

  - Depleting natural resources

  - World population growth

© 2008 Jones and Bartlett Publishers, Inc. (www.jbpub.com)

Notes

_____

Community Health in the Early 2000s - 4

- **Lifestyle Diseases**
  - Leading cause of death

  - Increase in obesity

  - Better control of behavioral risk factors, e.g., poor diet, inactivity, smoking, abuse of alcohol & drugs

© 2008 Jones and Bartlett Publishers, Inc. (www.jbpub.com)

Community Health in the Early 2000s - 5

- **Communicable Diseases**
  - Morbidity

  - Re-emerging, emerging, and drug-resistant diseases

  - Crossover diseases from animals

  - Use of pathogens for terrorism

© 2008 Jones and Bartlett Publishers, Inc. (www.jbpub.com)

Community Health in the Early 2000s - 6

- **Alcohol and Other Drug Abuse**
  - Costs: lives and money

  - Associated with unintentional injuries, domestic violence, and violent crimes

  - Many trying to deal with the problem

© 2008 Jones and Bartlett Publishers, Inc. (www.jbpub.com)

Community Health in the Early 2000s - 7

- **Disasters**
  - Natural: floods, hurricanes, earthquakes

  - Humanmade: unintentional (e.g., spill of toxic substance), & intentional (e.g., bioterrorism)

  - Lack of preparedness

  - DHS, DHHS, & CDC

© 2008 Jones and Bartlett Publishers, Inc. (www.jbpub.com)

Outlook for Community Health in the 21st Century

- **World Planning**
  - "Health for All"
  - Some progress
  - Widening gap between developed and undeveloped
  - Much work to be done: chronic noncommunicable diseases, traffic incidents
  - *United Nations Millennium Declaration*

© 2008 Jones and Bartlett Publishers, Inc. (www.jbpub.com)

HEALTHY PEOPLE

- The nation's health promotion and disease prevention agenda

- A roadmap to improve health using a 10-year plan

- Comprises three parts

© 2008 Jones and Bartlett Publishers, Inc. (www.jbpub.com)

Notes

Healthy People - 2

- **Part I**
  Understanding & Improving Health
  - History
  - Determinants of health model
  - How to use a systematic approach
  - Leading Health Indicators (LHI)

Healthy People - 3

- *Part II – Healthy People 2010: Objectives for Improving Health*
  - Overarching goals
    - Increase quality and years of healthy life
    - Eliminate health disparities
  - 467 objectives distributed over 28 focus areas
- Part III – *Tracking Healthy People 2010*
  - provides a comprehensive review of the statistical measures that will be used to evaluate progress

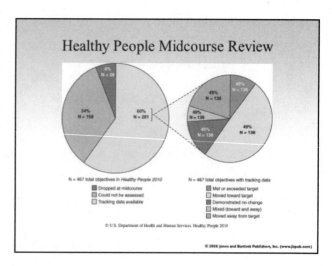

Healthy People Midcourse Review

Notes

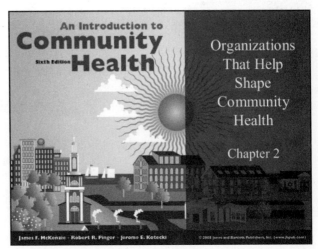

Introduction - 1

- **Today's Communities**
  - More educated, mobile, and more independent than past communities

  - In need of better long-term planning and community organizing due to large size of today's communities

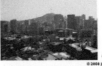

© Photos.com

© 2008 Jones and Bartlett Publishers, Inc. (www.jbpub.com)

Introduction - 2

- **Today's communities' ability to respond to their own problems is hindered by:**
  - Highly developed and centralized resources at national level
  - Continued concentration of wealth and population in the largest metropolitan areas
  - Rapid movement of information, resources, and people
  - Globalization of health
  - Limited horizontal relationships among organizations
  - Top-down funding for many community programs

© 2008 Jones and Bartlett Publishers, Inc. (www.jbpub.com)

Classification of Community Organizations

- **Classified by: sources of funding, responsibilities, & organizational structure**
- **Major types–**
  - Governmental
  - Quasi-governmental
  - Nongovernmental

© 2008 Jones and Bartlett Publishers, Inc. (www.jbpub.com)

Governmental Health Agencies

- Funded primarily by tax dollars
- Managed by government officials
- Authority for some geographic area
- Found at several levels
  - International, e.g., WHO
  - National, e.g., DHHS
  - State, e.g., Indiana Department of Health
  - Local, e.g., Delaware County Health Department

© 2008 Jones and Bartlett Publishers, Inc. (www.jbpub.com)

World Health Organization - 1

- **History**
  - United Nations charter in 1945 established need
  - Began April 7, 1948—World Health Day

- **Organization**
  - Membership open to countries that ratify constitution
  - Headquartered in Geneva, Switzerland
  - World Health Assembly; comprised of 193 delegates
  - Administered by director-general and 9 assistant directors-general

© 2008 Jones and Bartlett Publishers, Inc. (www.jbpub.com)

World Health Organization - 2

- **Purpose**
  - Attainment by all peoples of the highest possible level of health
- **Work**
  - Guided by *General Programme of Work* and *United Nations Millennium Declaration*
  - Most work carried out in poor countries
- **Millennium Development Goals (MDGs)**
  - 1) strengthening health systems; 2) ensuring health is a priority; 3) address the diverse needs of countries; 4) mobilizing more resources for health in poor countries; 5) improving health-related data

© 2008 Jones and Bartlett Publishers, Inc. (www.jbpub.com)

National Health Agencies

- **All countries have a primary department or agency responsible for the health of the citizens**
- **Department of Health & Human Services**
  - Principal agency for protecting the health of all Americans and providing essential human services
- **Other agencies also contribute to nation's health**
  - Examples: U.S. Dept. of Agriculture (includes WIC program); Occupational Safety and Health Administration (OSHA); Environmental Protection Agency (EPA)

© 2008 Jones and Bartlett Publishers, Inc. (www.jbpub.com)

Department of Health & Human Services - 1

© U.S. Department of Health and Human Services

© 2008 Jones and Bartlett Publishers, Inc. (www.jbpub.com)

Notes

_____
_____
_____
_____
_____
_____
_____
_____
_____
_____
_____
_____
_____
_____
_____
_____
_____
_____
_____
_____
_____
_____
_____
_____
_____
_____
_____
_____
_____
_____
_____
_____
_____
_____
_____
_____

Department of Health & Human Services - 2

- **Largest department in federal government; 25% of annual federal budget**

- **Organization**
  - Secretary of HHS
  - 11 agencies
  - 10 Regional offices

© 2008 Jones and Bartlett Publishers, Inc. (www.jbpub.com)

Agencies of HHS - 1

- **Administration on Aging (AoA)**– Designated to carry out the provisions of the Older Americans Act of 1965

- **Administration for Children and Families (ACF)**– Responsible for providing direction and leadership for all federal programs for needy children and families (administers Head Start program)

© 2008 Jones and Bartlett Publishers, Inc. (www.jbpub.com)

Agencies of HHS - 2

- **Agency for Healthcare Research and Quality (AHRQ)**– Lead federal agency for research on health care quality, costs, outcomes, and patient safety

- **Agency for Toxic Substances and Disease Registry (ATSDR)**– created by Superfund legislation; serves public to prevent harmful exposures and diseases related to toxic substances

© 2008 Jones and Bartlett Publishers, Inc. (www.jbpub.com)

Agencies of HHS - 3

- **Centers for Disease Control and Prevention (CDC)**– The nation's premiere health promotion, prevention, and preparedness agency and global leader in public health

- **Food and Drug Administration (FDA)**– Responsible for protecting the public health by assuring the safety, efficacy, and security of human and veterinary drugs, biological products, medical devices, food supply, cosmetics, and products that emit radiation

© 2008 Jones and Bartlett Publishers, Inc. (www.jbpub.com)

Agencies of HHS - 4

- **Centers for Medicare and Medicaid Services (CMS)**– Administers the Medicare (elderly & certain disabilities) & Medicaid (poor) programs which provide health care coverage to about 87 million Americans

- **Health Resources and Services Administration (HRSA)**– Helps provide health resources for medically underserved populations; works to build the health care workforce

© 2008 Jones and Bartlett Publishers, Inc. (www.jbpub.com)

Agencies of HHS - 5

- **Indian Health Services (IHS)**– Has the goal to raise physical, mental, social, and spiritual health of American Indians and Alaskan Natives to the highest level

- **Substance Abuse and Mental Health Services Administration (SAMHSA)**– Ensures up-to-date information and state-of-the-art practice is effectively used for the prevention and treatment of addictive and mental disorders

© 2008 Jones and Bartlett Publishers, Inc. (www.jbpub.com)

Notes

_____
_____
_____
_____
_____
_____
_____
_____
_____
_____
_____
_____
_____
_____
_____
_____
_____
_____
_____
_____
_____
_____
_____
_____
_____
_____
_____
_____
_____
_____
_____
_____
_____

Agencies of HHS - 6

- **National Institutes of Health (NIH)–**
  - One of the world's foremost medical research centers and the federal focal point for medical research in the U.S.

  - Examples: National Cancer Institute (NCI); National Heart, Lung, and Blood Institute (NHLBI); National Human Genome Research Institute (NHGRI)

© 2008 Jones and Bartlett Publishers, Inc. (www.jbpub.com)

State Health Agencies - 1

- **Every state has a state department of health**

- **Purpose**
  - To promote, protect, and maintain the health and welfare of their citizens

- **Core Functions of Public Health**
  - Assessment
  - Policy development
  - Assurance

© 2008 Jones and Bartlett Publishers, Inc. (www.jbpub.com)

State Health Agencies - 2

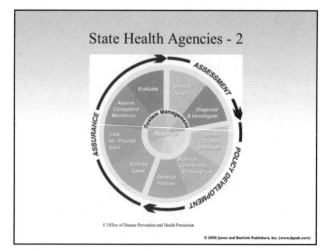

© Office of Disease Prevention and Health Promotion

© 2008 Jones and Bartlett Publishers, Inc. (www.jbpub.com)

State Health Agencies - 3

Typical Bureaus or Divisions

- Administration
- Communicable Disease Prevention & Control
- Chronic Disease Prevention & Control
- Vital & Health Statistics
- Health Education or Promotion
- Mental Health

- Maternal & Child Health
- Occupational & Industrial Health
- Dental Health
- Laboratory Services
- Public Health Nursing
- Veterinary Public Health

© 2008 Jones and Bartlett Publishers, Inc. (www.jbpub.com)

Local Health Departments - 1

- Responsibility of city or county governments; funded by tax dollars, grant dollars, & fees (sliding scale)

- Almost 3,000 nationwide; 62% in non-metropolitan areas & 38% in metropolitan areas

- Many services mandated by state laws; examples: restaurant inspections, reporting of certain communicable diseases, birth & death certificates

© 2008 Jones and Bartlett Publishers, Inc. (www.jbpub.com)

Local Health Departments - 2

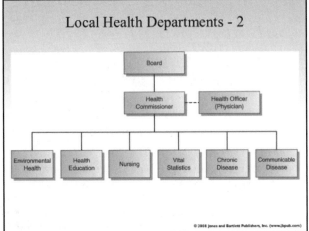

© 2008 Jones and Bartlett Publishers, Inc. (www.jbpub.com)

Notes

Coordinated School Health Program

- **Defined**
  - An organized set of policies, procedures, and activities designed to protect, promote, and improve the health and well-being of students and staff, thus improving the student's ability to learn.

- **Has great potential for improving health**

- **Many barriers**

© 2008 Jones and Bartlett Publishers, Inc. (www.jbpub.com)

Barriers to Coordinated School Health Programs

1. **Insufficient local administrative support**
2. **Inadequately prepared teachers**
3. **Too few school days to teach in the school year**
4. **Inadequate funding**
5. **Lack of credibility of health education as an academic subject**
6. **Insufficient community/parental support**
7. **Concern for the teaching of controversial topics (i.e., sex education)**

© 2008 Jones and Bartlett Publishers, Inc. (www.jbpub.com)

Quasi-governmental Organizations

- **Some responsibilities assigned by government but operate more like voluntary agencies**
- **Funded by tax dollars & private sources**
- **Operate independently of government supervision**
- **Examples: American Red Cross, National Academy of Science**

© 2008 Jones and Bartlett Publishers, Inc. (www.jbpub.com)

Notes

American Red Cross

- **Founded in 1881 by Clara Barton**
- **"Official" Duties**
  - Provide relief to victims of natural disasters
  - Serve as a liaison between members of the active military and their families during emergencies
- **Nongovernmental services**
  - Blood drives, safety services, nursing and health services, youth services, community volunteer services, and international services

© 2008 Jones and Bartlett Publishers, Inc. (www.jbpub.com)

Nongovernmental Health Agencies

- **Funded by private donations or, in some cases, membership fees**

- **Free from governmental interference as long as they meet IRS guidelines**

- **Many types: voluntary, professional, social, philanthropic, service, religious, & corporate**

© 2008 Jones and Bartlett Publishers, Inc. (www.jbpub.com)

Voluntary Health Agencies

- **Created to meet a specific health need**

- **Basic objectives: research, education, services, advocacy**

- **Funded by donations; fundraising events**

- **Examples: ACS, AHA, ALA – big three**

© 2008 Jones and Bartlett Publishers, Inc. (www.jbpub.com)

Notes

Other Nongovernmental Health Agencies - 1

- **Professional Health Organizations/Associations**
  - Purpose: Promote high standards of professional practice for their specific profession
  - Examples: American Public Health Association, American Medical Association, American Nursing Association, Society for Public Health Education

- **Philanthropic Foundations**
  - Provide grants to support programs
  - Example: Bill and Melinda Gates Foundation

© 2008 Jones and Bartlett Publishers, Inc. (www.jbpub.com)

Other Nongovernmental Health Agencies - 2

- **Service, Social, & Religious Organization**
  - Most provide service & many sponsor health-related programs, i.e., "Lion's Quest," burn centers, food banks, sleeping rooms

- **Corporate America**
  - Workplace health & safety
  - Health insurance
  - Workplace health promotion

© 2008 Jones and Bartlett Publishers, Inc. (www.jbpub.com)

Chapter 3: Epidemiology: The Study of Disease, Injury, and Death in the Community

Notes

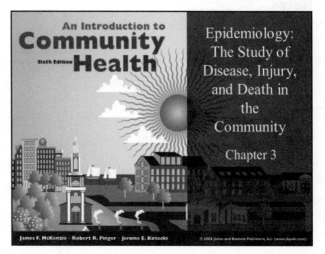

Introduction

- **An epidemiologist is to a population as a doctor is to a patient**
- **Study outbreaks of disease, injury, & death in the human population**
- **Questions asked by epidemiologists:** How many are sick? Who is sick? When did they get sick? Where did they get sick? What do the sick have in common?
- **Epidemiology has been called "population medicine"**

© 2008 Jones and Bartlett Publishers, Inc. (www.jbpub.com)

Definitions - 1

- **Epidemiology**– "the study of the distribution and determinants of health-related states or events in specified populations, and the application of this study to control health problems" (Last, 2001)
- **Endemic Diseases**– diseases that occur regularly in a population as a matter of course
- **Epidemic**– An unexpectedly large number of cases of an illness, specific health-related behavior, or other health-related event in a particular population

© 2008 Jones and Bartlett Publishers, Inc. (www.jbpub.com)

Recent Epidemics in the United States

Table 3.1
Recent Epidemics in the United States

Disease	Cases in Previous Years	Epidemic Period	Number of Cases
St. Louis encephalitis	5–72	1975	1,815 [?]
Legionnaires' disease	Unknown	1976	235 [?]
Toxic shock syndrome	11–272	1980	877 [?]
HIV/AIDS	Unknown	1981–2004	944,305 [?]
Lyme disease	Unknown	1990–2004	222,350 [?]
Plague	13–19	1983	40 [?]
West Nile virus	Unknown	1999–2005	18,756 [?]
Mumps	251–314	2006	5,423 [?]

© 2008 Jones and Bartlett Publishers, Inc. (www.jbpub.com)

Definitions - 2

- **Epidemiologist**– "an investigator who studies the occurrence of disease or other health-related conditions or events in defined populations" (Last, 2001)
- **Epizootic**– outbreak of disease that begins in animals and spreads to humans
- **Pandemic**– outbreak of disease over a wide geographical area such as a continent (flu pandemic of 1918-19 killed 25 million people worldwide)

© 2008 Jones and Bartlett Publishers, Inc. (www.jbpub.com)

Brief History of Epidemiology

- **300 *B.C.*: Hippocrates, "Father of Medicine,"** suggested a relationship between disease & environment
- **After fall of Greece & Rome, there were few advancements in health & medicine, & diseases became linked to spiritual causes**
- **1793: Yellow fever in Philadelphia;** killed 4,044 people; cause (mosquito) discovered in 1901 by Major Walter Reed
- **1849: Cholera in London;** Snow investigated & in 1854 removed Broad Street pump handle; 30 years before Louis Pasteur's "germ theory"

© 2008 Jones and Bartlett Publishers, Inc. (www.jbpub.com)

The Importance of Rates

- **Cases**– those afflicted

- **Rates**– the number of events that occur in a given population in a given period of time; three categories– natality (birth), morbidity (sickness), & mortality or fatality (death) rates

- **Importance of Rates**– allows for a comparison of outbreaks that occur at different times or in different places

Rates Defined

- **Incidence rate**– the number of new health-related events or cases of a disease in a population exposed to that risk in a given time period

- **Prevalence rate**– calculated by dividing *all* current cases of a disease (*old* & *new*) by the total population

- **Attack rate**– a special incidence rate calculated for a particular population for a single disease outbreak expressed as a percentage

Definitions associated with Incidence, Prevalence, & Attack Rates

- **Acute diseases**– those that last three months or less

- **Chronic diseases**– those that last three months or longer

Notes

Incidence, Prevalence, & Attack Rates

Table 3.3
Incidence Rates, Prevalence Rates, and Attack Rates

Name of Rate		Definition of Rate	
Incidence rate	=	$\dfrac{\text{Number of new health-related events or cases of a disease}}{\text{Number of people exposed to risk during this period}}$	
Prevalence rate	=	$\dfrac{\text{Total number of all individuals who have an attribute or disease at a time}}{\text{Population at risk of having the attribute or disease at this point or period of time}}$	
Attack rate*	=	$\dfrac{\text{The cumulative incidence of infection in a group observed during an epidemic}}{\text{Number of people exposed}}$	× 100

*Attack rates are usually given as a percentage.

© 2008 Jones and Bartlett Publishers, Inc. (www.jbpub.com)

Crude, Age-Adjusted, & Specific Rates

- **Crude rates**– those in which the dominator includes the total population

- **Age-adjusted rates**– those used to make comparisons of relative risks across group & over time when groups differ in age structure

- **Specific rates**– measure morbidity or mortality for particular populations or diseases

© 2008 Jones and Bartlett Publishers, Inc. (www.jbpub.com)

Important Rates in Epidemiology

Table 3.6
Important Rates in Epidemiology

Rate		Definition	Multiplier	Examples (U.S. 2004)ᵃ⁻ᶜ
Crude birth rate	=	$\dfrac{\text{Number of live births}}{\text{Estimated midyear population}}$	× 1,000	14.0/1000
Crude death rate	=	$\dfrac{\text{Number of deaths (all causes)}}{\text{Estimated midyear population}}$	× 1,000	8.0/1000
Age-specific death rate	=	$\dfrac{\text{Number of deaths, 15–24}}{\text{Estimated midyear population, 15–24}}$	× 100,000	79.2/100,000
Infant mortality rate	=	$\dfrac{\text{Number of deaths under 1 year of age}}{\text{Number of live births}}$	× 100,000	6.76/1000
Neonatal mortality rate	=	$\dfrac{\text{Number of deaths under 28 days of age}}{\text{Number of live births}}$	× 100,000	4.5/1000
Cause-specific death rate	=	$\dfrac{\text{Number of deaths (diabetes mellitus)}}{\text{Estimated midyear population}}$	× 100,000	24.8/100,000
Age-specific, cause-specific death rate	=	$\dfrac{\text{Number of deaths, 15–24 (motor vehicles)}}{\text{Estimated midyear population}}$	× 100,000	26.1/100,000

© 2008 Jones and Bartlett Publishers, Inc. (www.jbpub.com)

Reporting of Births, Deaths, & Diseases

- **Notifiable diseases**– infectious diseases which health officials request or require reporting

- **National Electronic Telecommunications System (NETS)**– the electronic reporting system used by state health departments and CDC

- *Morbidity and Mortality Weekly Report (MMWR)*– a report of CDC used to present notifiable disease data

© 2008 Jones and Bartlett Publishers, Inc. (www.jbpub.com)

Scheme for the Reporting of Notifiable Diseases

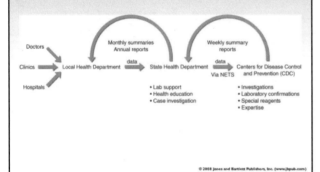

© 2008 Jones and Bartlett Publishers, Inc. (www.jbpub.com)

Standardized Measurements of Health Status of Populations - 1

- **Mortality statistics**– single most reliable measure of population health
  - 1900: Pneumonia & influenza, TB, diarrhea
  - 2004: Heart disease, cancer, stroke

- **Life expectancy**– average number of years a person from a specific cohort (e.g., born in 2008) is projected to live from a given point in time (e.g., birth, age 65, age 75)

© 2008 Jones and Bartlett Publishers, Inc. (www.jbpub.com)

Notes

Life Expectancy at Birth, 65, and 75

Table 3.10
Life Expectancy at Birth, at 65 Years of Age, and at 75 Years of Age According to Sex:
In the United States, During the Selected Years 1900–2003

	At Birth			At 65 Years			At 75 Years		
Year	Both Sexes	Male	Female	Both Sexes	Male	Female	Both Sexes	Male	Female
1900	47.3	46.3	48.3	11.9	11.5	12.2	*	*	*
1950	68.2	65.6	71.1	13.9	12.8	15.0	*	*	*
1960	69.7	66.6	73.1	14.3	12.8	15.8	*	*	*
1970	70.8	67.1	74.7	15.2	13.1	17.0	*	*	*
1980	73.7	70.7	77.4	16.4	14.1	18.3	10.4	8.8	11.5
1990	75.4	71.8	78.8	17.2	15.1	18.9	10.9	9.4	12.0
2003	77.5	74.8	80.1	18.4	16.8	19.8	11.8	10.5	12.6

*Data not available.

Source: Adapted from the National Center for Health Statistics (2006). *Health, United States, 2006 with Chartbook on Trends in the Health of Americans.* (DHHS pub. no. 2006-1252). Hyattsville, MD: Public Health Service.

© 2008 Jones and Bartlett Publishers, Inc. (www.jbpub.com)

Standardized Measurements of Health Status of Populations - 2

- **Years of potential life lost (YPLL)**– number of years lost when death occurs before age 65 or 75
- **Disability-adjusted life years (DALYs)**– measure of the burden of disease that takes into account premature death & loss of healthy life resulting from disability
- **Health-adjusted life expectancy (HALE)**– number of years of healthy life expected on average in a given population

© 2008 Jones and Bartlett Publishers, Inc. (www.jbpub.com)

Sources of Standardized Data -1

- **U.S. Census**– Conducted every 10 years; enumeration of population

- *Statistical Abstract of the United States*– a book published annually that includes statistics on social, political, and economic organization

- *Monthly Vital Statistics Report*– Statistical summaries of records of major life events

© 2008 Jones and Bartlett Publishers, Inc. (www.jbpub.com)

Sources of Standardized Data - 2

- *Morbidity & Mortality Weekly Report* (MMWR)– Prepared by the CDC & reports cases of notifiable diseases in the U.S.; also includes articles on other public health problems
- **National Health Surveys**
  - Many different ones; most conducted by NCHS or CDC
  - Better known: NHIS (questions about health); NHANES (health & nutritional status using mobile van); BRFSS & YRBSS (behavior risk factors); NHCS (health care)

© 2008 Jones and Bartlett Publishers, Inc. (www.jbpub.com)

Epidemiological Studies - 1

- **Descriptive Studies**
  - Who (or person): Age, sex, ethnic, race, socioeconomic status
  - When (or time): Time of day, week, month, season, year, decades; incubation period
  - Where (or place): Country, state, county, street, urban or rural, domestic or foreign, institutional or non-institutional

© 2008 Jones and Bartlett Publishers, Inc. (www.jbpub.com)

Epidemiological Studies - 2

- **To answer the question of– When?**
  - Epidemic curve: a graphic display of the cases of a disease according to the time or date of onset
  - Point source epidemic: an epidemic curve depicting a distribution of cases which all can be traced to a single source
  - Propagated epidemic curve: an epidemic curve depicting a distribution of cases traceable to multiple sources of exposure

© 2008 Jones and Bartlett Publishers, Inc. (www.jbpub.com)

Notes

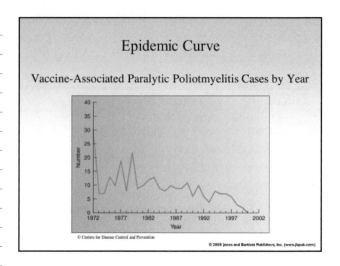

Epidemic Curve

Vaccine-Associated Paralytic Poliotmyelitis Cases by Year

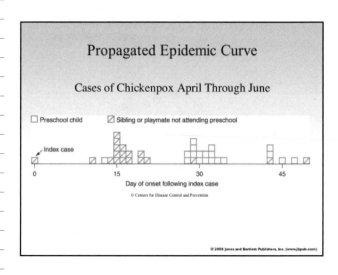

Propagated Epidemic Curve

Cases of Chickenpox April Through June

Epidemiological Studies - 3

- **Analytical Studies**
  - Purpose: testing of hypotheses about relationships between health problems and possible risk factors
  - Two basic types: observational and experimental studies
  - Observational

Epidemiological Studies - 4

- **Analytical Studies (continued)–**
  - Experimental (interventional)
    - Case/control study (retrospective): one that seeks to compare those diagnosed with a disease with those who do not have the disease for prior exposure to specific risk factors
    - Cohort study (prospective study): one in which a cohort is classified by exposure to one or more specific risk factors and observed to determine the rates at which disease develops in each group

© 2008 Jones and Bartlett Publishers, Inc. (www.jbpub.com)

Epidemiological Studies - 5

- **Other key terms–**
  - Odds ratio: a probability statement about the association between a particular disease & specific risk factor resulting from a case/control study

  - Relative risk: a statement of the relationship between the risk of acquiring a disease when a specific risk factor is present and the risk of acquiring that same disease when the risk factor is absent

  - Placebo: a blank treatment

© 2008 Jones and Bartlett Publishers, Inc. (www.jbpub.com)

Notes

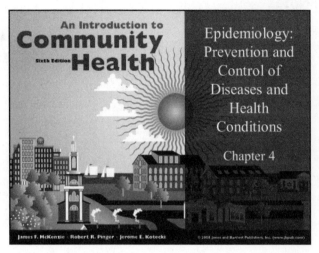

Classification of Diseases & Health Problems

- **Communicable (infectious) vs. Noncommunicable (noninfectious) Diseases**
  - Communicable: caused by specific biological agent or its product and can be transmitted from infected to susceptible host
  - Noncommunicable: one that cannot be transmitted from infected to susceptible host
- **Acute vs. Chronic Diseases & Illnesses**
  - Acute: last 3 months or less
  - Chronic: last more than 3 months

© 2008 Jones and Bartlett Publishers, Inc. (www.jbpub.com)

Causative Agents for Diseases & Injuries

Table 4.1
Causative Agents for Diseases and Injuries

Biological Agents	Chemical Agents	Physical Agents
Viruses	Pesticides	Heat
Rickettsiae	Food additives	Light
Bacteria	Pharmacologics	Radiation
Fungi	Industrial chemicals	Noise
Protozoa	Air pollutants	Vibration
Metazoa	Cigarette smoke	Speeding objects

© 2008 Jones and Bartlett Publishers, Inc. (www.jbpub.com)

Notes

Classification of Diseases

Table 4.2
Classification of Diseases

Types of Diseases	Examples
Acute diseases	
Communicable	Common cold, pneumonia, mumps, measles, pertussis, typhoid fever, cholera
Noncommunicable	Appendicitis, poisoning, injury (due to motor vehicle crash, fire, gunshot, etc.)
Chronic diseases	
Communicable	AIDS, Lyme disease, tuberculosis, syphilis, rheumatic fever following streptococcal infections, hepatitis B
Noncommunicable	Diabetes, coronary heart disease, osteoarthritis, cirrhosis of the liver due to alcoholism

© 2008 Jones and Bartlett Publishers, Inc. (www.jbpub.com)

Communicable Diseases

- **Key terms**
  - Infectivity: the ability of a biological agent to enter and grow in a host
  - Pathogenicity: the capability of a communicable disease agent to cause disease in a susceptible host
- **Communicable disease model**

Host

Agent / Environment

© 2008 Jones and Bartlett Publishers, Inc. (www.jbpub.com)

Communicable Disease Model - 1

Agent– the element that must be present in order for cause of the disease to occur

© 2008 Jones and Bartlett Publishers, Inc. (www.jbpub.com)

Communicable Disease Model - 2

Host– Any susceptible organism invaded by an infectious agent

Agent

© 2008 Jones and Bartlett Publishers, Inc. (www.jbpub.com)

Communicable Disease Model - 3

Host

Agent

Environment– All other factors that inhibit or promote disease transmission

© 2008 Jones and Bartlett Publishers, Inc. (www.jbpub.com)

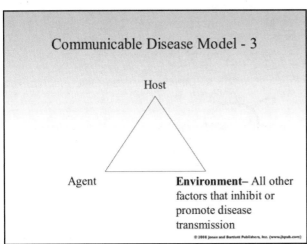

Chain of Infection - 1

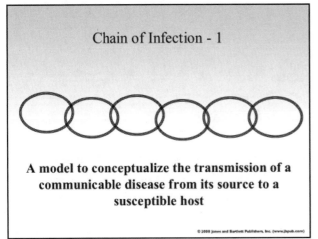

A model to conceptualize the transmission of a communicable disease from its source to a susceptible host

© 2008 Jones and Bartlett Publishers, Inc. (www.jbpub.com)

Notes

Notes

Chain of Infection - 2

- **Pathogen**– the disease-causing agent (e.g., virus, bacteria, rickettsiae, protozoa, fungi & yeasts, nematoda)

Chain of Infection - 3

- **Reservoir**– the habitat in which an infectious agent normally lives & grows
  - Human: Anthroponoses; symptomatic or asymptomatic
  - Animal: Zoonoses
  - Environmental: Plants, soil, & water

Chain of Infection - 4

- **Portal of exit**– the path by which an agent leaves the source host

Chain of Infection - 5

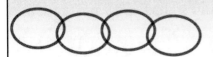

- **Modes of Transmission– how pathogens are passed**
  - Direct (immediate transfer): direct contact, droplet spread
  - Indirect: airborne, vehicleborne, vectorborne (mechanical & biological)

© 2008 Jones and Bartlett Publishers, Inc. (www.jbpub.com)

Chain of Infection - 6

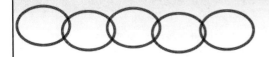

- **Portal of entry**– agent enters susceptible host; means (respiratory, oral, skin, intravenous, gastrointestinal)

© 2008 Jones and Bartlett Publishers, Inc. (www.jbpub.com)

Chain of Infection - 7

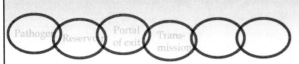

- **New host**– final link is a susceptible host

© 2008 Jones and Bartlett Publishers, Inc. (www.jbpub.com)

Notes

Notes

_____

Chain of Infection - 8

Reservoir   Transmission   Establishment

Pathogen   Portal of entry   Portal of exit

© 2008 Jones and Bartlett Publishers, Inc. (www.jbpub.com)

Noncommunicable Diseases

- **Complex etiologies (causes)**

- **Multicausation disease model**
  – Genetics
  – Personality & beliefs
  – Behavioral choices
  – Environment

© 2008 Jones and Bartlett Publishers, Inc. (www.jbpub.com)

Multicausation Disease Model - 1

Your genetic endowment

© 2008 Jones and Bartlett Publishers, Inc. (www.jbpub.com)

Multicausation Disease Model - 2

Personality

Beliefs

Your genetic endowment

Behavioral choices

© 2008 Jones and Bartlett Publishers, Inc. (www.jbpub.com)

Multicausation Disease Model - 3

Environment

Your personality, beliefs, and behavioral choices

Economics

Health care system

Your genetic endowment

Air pollution

Water quality

Infectious disease outbreaks

© 2008 Jones and Bartlett Publishers, Inc. (www.jbpub.com)

Diseases of the Heart & Blood (Cardiovascular Diseases [CVD])

- **Coronary heart disease** (CHD)– Characterized by damage to the coronary arteries; also called coronary artery disease; #1 killer

- **Atherosclerosis**– Narrowing of the blood vessels resulting from the build-up of fatty deposits on the walls of the blood vessel

- **Cerebrovascular disease** (stroke)– Blood supply to the brain is disrupted; #3 killer

© 2008 Jones and Bartlett Publishers, Inc. (www.jbpub.com)

Notes

Malignant Neoplasms (Cancer)

- **Cancer**– occurs when cells lose control over their growth and division; develop into a tumor; #2 killer

- **Metastasis**– parts of the tumor break off & travel to the rest of the body's organs and continue their growth

- **Stages**– I, II, III, & IV; most curable in early stages

© 2008 Jones and Bartlett Publishers, Inc. (www.jbpub.com)

Other Noncommunicable Disease Problems

- **Chronic obstructive pulmonary disease (COPD)**– #4 killer

- **Diabetes mellitus**– #7 killer

- **Chronic liver disease and cirrhosis**– #10 killer

© 2008 Jones and Bartlett Publishers, Inc. (www.jbpub.com)

Prioritizing Prevention & Control Efforts

- **Leading causes of death**– CHD, cancer, stroke

- **Years of potential life lost**– cancer, CHD, unintentional injuries

- **Economic cost to society**– alcohol and other drugs

© 2008 Jones and Bartlett Publishers, Inc. (www.jbpub.com)

Prevention, Intervention, Control, & Eradication of Diseases

- **Prevention**– the planning for & taking of action to forestall the onset of a disease or other health problem (e.g., immunization)
- **Intervention**– taking action during an event (e.g., taking an antibiotic)
- **Control**– containment of disease; limiting transmission
- **Eradication**– total elimination of the disease

© AbleStock

© 2008 Jones and Bartlett Publishers, Inc. (www.jbpub.com)

Levels of Prevention

- **Primary Prevention**– measures that forestall the onset of illness or injury during the pre-pathogenesis period (e.g., immunizations)
- **Secondary Prevention**– measures that lead to early diagnosis & prompt treatment of a disease or injury to limit disability or prevent more severe pathogenesis (e.g., screenings)
- **Tertiary Prevention**– measures aimed at rehabilitation following significant pathogenesis (e.g., physical therapy)

© 2008 Jones and Bartlett Publishers, Inc. (www.jbpub.com)

Prevention of Communicable Diseases

Pathogen	Human reservoir	Portal of exit	Transmission	Portal of entry	Establishment of disease in new host
• Pasteurization	• Isolation	• Gowns	• Isolation	• Masks	• Immunizations
• Chlorination	• Surveillance	• Masks	• Hand washing	• Condoms	• Health education
• Antibiotics	• Quarantine	• Condoms	• Vector control	• Safety glasses	• Nutrition promotion
• Antivirals	• Drug treatment	• Hair nets	• Sanitary engineering	• Insect repellents	• Sexual abstinence
• Disinfectants		• Insect repellents	• Sneeze glass		
			• Sexual abstinence		
			• Safe sex		

© 2008 Jones and Bartlett Publishers, Inc. (www.jbpub.com)

Notes

Notes

Prevention of Noncommunicable Diseases -1

- **Primary Prevention**
  - Good health behavior (eating properly, exercising adequately, etc.)
  - Community health & medical services
  - Health education & promotion programs
  - Access to medical services
  - Protection from environmental & occupational hazards
  - Empowerment for one's own health

© 2008 Jones and Bartlett Publishers, Inc. (www.jbpub.com)

Prevention of Noncommunicable Diseases - 2

- **Secondary Prevention**
  - Mass screenings (blood pressure, cholesterol, etc.)
  - Case-finding measures (STDs, TB, etc.)
  - Adequate health personnel, equipment, and facilities
  - Personal screening (self-breast & testicular exams)
  - Cancer screenings (hemoccult tests, Pap tests, PSAs, etc.)

© 2008 Jones and Bartlett Publishers, Inc. (www.jbpub.com)

Prevention of Noncommunicable Diseases - 3

- **Tertiary Prevention**
  - Adequate emergency medical personnel, services, and facilities
  - Understand unmodifiable risk factors
  - Significant behavioral or lifestyle changes of modifiable risk factors
  - Rehab programs (e.g., cardiac rehab)
  - Support groups
  - Counseling

© 2008 Jones and Bartlett Publishers, Inc. (www.jbpub.com)

Chapter 5: Community Organizing/Building and Health Promotion Programming

Notes

_____

_____

_____

_____

_____

_____

_____

_____

_____

_____

_____

_____

_____

_____

_____

_____

_____

_____

_____

_____

_____

_____

_____

_____

_____

_____

_____

_____

_____

_____

_____

_____

_____

_____

_____

_____

_____

_____

_____

_____

An Introduction to Community Health

Sixth Edition

Community Organizing/ Building and Health Promotion Programming

Chapter 5

James F. McKenzie · Robert R. Pinger · Jerome E. Kotecki

© 2008 Jones and Bartlett Publishers, Inc. (www.jbpub.com)

Introduction

- **Epidemiology important to community health**

- **Two other skills for community health workers**
  - Community organizing/building
  - Health promotion programming

© 2008 Jones and Bartlett Publishers, Inc. (www.jbpub.com)

Community Organizing Defined

"A process through which communities are helped to identify common problems or goals, mobilize resources, and in other ways develop and implement strategies for reaching their goals they have collectively set" (Minkler & Wallerstein, 2005)

© 2008 Jones and Bartlett Publishers, Inc. (www.jbpub.com)

Notes

Related Definitions - 1

- **Community capacity**– Community characteristics affecting its ability to identify, mobilize, & address problems (Goodman et al., 1999)

- **Empowered community**– "One in which individuals and organizations apply their skills and resources in collective efforts to meet their respective needs" (Israel et al., 1994)

© 2008 Jones and Bartlett Publishers, Inc. (www.jbpub.com)

Related Definitions - 2

- **Participation & relevance**– "Community organizing that starts where the people are and engages community members as equals" (Minkler & Wallerstein, 2005)

- **Social capital**– "relationships and structures within a community that promote cooperation for mutual benefit" (Minkler & Wallerstein, 2005)

© 2008 Jones and Bartlett Publishers, Inc. (www.jbpub.com)

Need for Organizing Communities

- **Advances have moved us to the need to organize**
  - Electronics (e.g., digital TV)
  - Communications (e.g., multi-function cell phones)
  - Household upgrades (e.g., energy efficiency)
  - Increased mobility (e.g., frequency of moving)
  - Lack of interaction with neighbors
  - Size of communities

© 2008 Jones and Bartlett Publishers, Inc. (www.jbpub.com)

Assumptions of Community Organization

1. Communities of people can develop the capacity to deal with their own problems
2. People want to change and can change
3. People should participate in making, adjusting, or controlling the major changes taking place within their communities
4. Changes in community living that are self-imposed or self-developed have a meaning and permanence that imposed changes do not have

© 2008 Jones and Bartlett Publishers, Inc. (www.jbpub.com)

Assumptions of Community Organization - 2

5. A "holistic approach" can deal successfully with problems with which a "fragmented approach" cannot cope
6. Democracy requires cooperative participation and action in the affairs of the community, and people must learn the skills that make this possible
7. Frequently, communities of people need help in organizing to deal with their needs, just as many individuals require help with individual problems

© 2008 Jones and Bartlett Publishers, Inc. (www.jbpub.com)

Community Organizing Methods

- **Locality development**– based on the concept of broad self-help participation from the local community

- **Social planning**– heavily task oriented, stressing rational-empirical problem solving, and involves various levels of participation from many people and outside planners

- **Social action**– a technique that involves the redistribution of power & resources to disadvantaged segments of the population

© 2008 Jones and Bartlett Publishers, Inc. (www.jbpub.com)

Generic Approach to Community Organizing - 1

- **Recognizing the issue**
  - From the inside– grass-roots, citizen initiated, bottom up
  - From the outside– top down

- **Gaining entry into the community**
  - Gatekeepers
  - Being culturally sensitive and working toward culturally competent

© 2008 Jones and Bartlett Publishers, Inc. (www.jbpub.com)

Generic Approach to Community Organizing - 2

- **Organizing the people**
  - Executive participants
  - Networking and expanding the constituencies
  - Creating an association, task force or coalition

- **Assessing the community**
  - Needs based vs. assets based; mapping
  - Community building: "an orientation to community that is strength-based rather than need-based and stresses the identification, nurturing, and celebration of community assets" (Minkler, 2005)

© 2008 Jones and Bartlett Publishers, Inc. (www.jbpub.com)

Generic Approach to Community Organizing - 3

- **Determining the priorities & setting goals**
  - Build ownership
  - Five criteria for selecting problem: winnable, simple & specific, must unite, affect many & build community, & part of larger plan (Miller)

- **Arriving at a solution & selecting intervention strategies**
  - Create an intervention
  - Avoid *turfism*

© 2008 Jones and Bartlett Publishers, Inc. (www.jbpub.com)

Generic Approach to Community Organizing - 4

The Final Four Steps

Implementing

Looping back

Evaluating

Maintaining

© 2008 Jones and Bartlett Publishers, Inc. (www.jbpub.com)

Other Models Used for Community Organizing/Building

- **Healthy Cities/Healthy Communities**
- **Mobilizing for Action through Planning & Partnerships (MAPP)**
- **Planned Approach to Community Health (PATCH)**

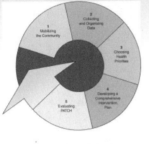

1 Mobilizing the Community
2 Collecting and Organizing Data
3 Choosing Health Priorities
4 Developing a Comprehensive Intervention Plan
5 Evaluating PATCH

© Centers for Disease Control and Prevention

© 2008 Jones and Bartlett Publishers, Inc. (www.jbpub.com)

Health Promotion Programming - 1

- **Health education**– "any combination of planned learning experiences based on sound theories that provide individuals, groups, and communities the opportunity to acquire information and the skills to make quality health decisions" (Joint Committee, 1991)

- **Health promotion**– "any planned combination of educational, political, environmental, regulatory, or organizational mechanisms that support actions and conditions of living conducive to health of individuals, groups, and communities" (Joint Committee, 1999)

© 2008 Jones and Bartlett Publishers, Inc. (www.jbpub.com)

Notes

Health Promotion Programming - 2

- **Many different planning models**
  - PRECEDE/PROCEED: best known
  - Multilevel Approach to Community Health (MATCH)
  - Intervention Mapping: newest model
  - CDCynergy: best for health communication
  - Social Marketing Assessment & Response Tool (SMART)
  - Generalized Model for Program Planning

Generalized Model for Program Planning - 1

- **Preliminary steps**
  - Who makes up the priority population?
  - Understand & engage the priority population
  - Planning committee

- **Assessing the Needs of the Priority Population**

Generalized Model for Program Planning - 2
Assessing the Needs

Determining the purpose & scope

Gathering data

Analyzing the data

Identifying factors linked to the health problem

Identifying the program focus

Validating the prioritized need

Notes

Generalized Model for Program Planning - 3

After the needs assessment should have answers to:

- Who is the priority population?
- What are the needs of the priority population?
- Which subgroups within the priority population have the greatest need?
- Where are the subgroups located geographically?
- What is currently being done to resolve identified needs?
- How well have the identified needs been addressed in the past?

© 2008 Jones and Bartlett Publishers, Inc. (www.jbpub.com)

Generalized Model for Program Planning - 4

- **Setting Appropriate Goals & Objectives**
  - Goals: future event
  - Objectives: steps to reach goals; several levels (process/administrative, learning, action/behavioral, environmental, program)

- **Creating an Intervention**
  - Activities to reach goals and objectives
  - Amount is important; multiple exposures
  - Consider ecological perspective; multiple levels

© 2008 Jones and Bartlett Publishers, Inc. (www.jbpub.com)

Generalized Model for Program Planning - 5

- **Implementing the Intervention**
  - Pilot test
  - Phasing in
  - Full implementation

- **Evaluating the Results**
  - The process of determining the value or worth of the object of interest
  - Standards of acceptability: stated in the objectives
  - Formative & summative

© 2008 Jones and Bartlett Publishers, Inc. (www.jbpub.com)

Notes

Generalized Model for Program Planning - 6

Evaluating the Results

Planning the evaluation

© 2008 Jones and Bartlett Publishers, Inc. (www.jbpub.com)

Generalized Model for Program Planning - 7

Evaluating the Results

Planning the evaluation

Collecting the data

© 2008 Jones and Bartlett Publishers, Inc. (www.jbpub.com)

Generalized Model for Program Planning - 8

Evaluating the Results

Planning the evaluation

Collecting the data

Analyzing the data

© 2008 Jones and Bartlett Publishers, Inc. (www.jbpub.com)

Generalized Model for Program Planning - 9
Evaluating the Results

Planning the evaluation

⬇

Collecting the data

⬇

Analyzing the data

⬇

Reporting results

Generalized Model for Program Planning - 10
Evaluating the Results - 5

Planning the evaluation

⬇

Collecting the data

⬇

Analyzing the data

⬇

Reporting results

⬇

Applying the results

Notes

Chapter 6: The School Health Program: A Component of Community Health

Notes

The School Health Program: A Component of Community Health

Chapter 6

Introduction

- **Important component of community health**

- **Has great potential**

- **All must pass through**

Coordinated School Health Defined

- **"An organized set of policies, procedures, and activities designed to protect, promote, and improve the health and well-being of students and staff, thus improving the student's ability to learn" (Joint Committee, 2001)**

Notes

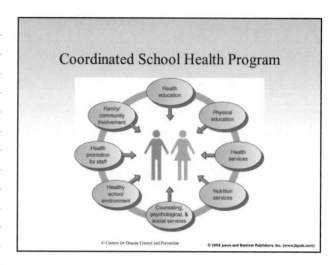

Coordinated School Health Program

School Health Council

Students   Parents

Teachers   Administrators

Medical personnel   Maintenance workers

Social workers   Food service workers

Counseling   Personnel

Primary role is to provide coordination of the various component of the CSHP

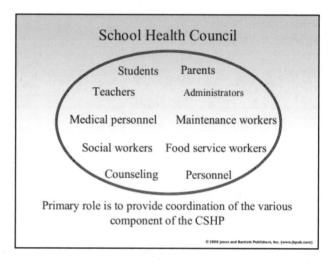

School Nurse

- Providing direct health care to students & staff
- Providing leadership for the provision of health services
- Providing screening & referral for health conditions
- Promoting a healthy school environment
- Promoting health
- Serving in a leadership role for health policies & programs
- Serving as a liaison between school personnel, family, community, & health care providers

Teachers' Role in CSHP

- **Instruction**

- **Observation of normal & abnormal**

- **Leadership & Coordination**

© 2008 Jones and Bartlett Publishers, Inc. (www.jbpub.com)

Need for School Health

- **Health of children and their learning are reciprocally related.**
  - Unhealthy child has a difficult time learning

  - Unhealthy child can be disruptive to others

  - School programs included in *Healthy People 2010*

  - Not a cure-all

© 2008 Jones and Bartlett Publishers, Inc. (www.jbpub.com)

Foundations of the School Health Program

| Support of school administration |
| Written school health policies |
| Well-organized school health council |

© 2008 Jones and Bartlett Publishers, Inc. (www.jbpub.com)

Notes

School Health Policies

- **Written statements that describe the nature & procedures of a school health program**
- **Policy development**– medical advisor, school administration, board of education
- **Policy implementation**– distribution & enforcement
- **Policy development resources**– wellness policies have helped; possible resources: *Action for Healthy Kids*, CDC, & ASCD

© 2008 Jones and Bartlett Publishers, Inc. (www.jbpub.com)

Components for CSHP - 1

- **Administration and Organization**
  - Supportive administration
  - School health coordinator
- **School Health Services**– health appraisals, emergency care services, prevention and control of communicable diseases, provisions for special needs students, health advising, remediation of detected health problems

© 2008 Jones and Bartlett Publishers, Inc. (www.jbpub.com)

Components for CSHP - 2

- **Healthy school environment**– the promotion, maintenance, and utilization of safe and wholesome surroundings in a school
  - Physical environment
  - Psychosocial environment

- **School health education**– the development, delivery, and evaluation of a planned curriculum, kindergarten through grade 12

© 2008 Jones and Bartlett Publishers, Inc. (www.jbpub.com)

Components for CSHP - 3

School Health Education

- **Curriculum**– written plan for school health education
  - Scope– what will be taught
  - Sequence– when it will be taught
- **Priority health content**– alcohol & drug-free lifestyle, healthy eating, mental & emotional health, personal health & wellness, physical activity, safety & injury prevention, sexual health, tobacco-free lifestyle, violence prevention

© 2008 Jones and Bartlett Publishers, Inc. (www.jbpub.com)

Components for CSHP - 4

- **Counseling, Psychological, & Social Services**– individual and group assessments, interventions, and referrals

- **Physical education**– "planned, sequential K-12 curriculum that provides cognitive content and learning experiences in a variety of activity areas" (DASH, 2005)

© 2008 Jones and Bartlett Publishers, Inc. (www.jbpub.com)

Components for CSHP - 5

- **School nutrition services**– nutritious and appealing meals; also nutrition education

- **Family/community involvement for school health**– "integrated school, parent, and community approach for enhancing the health and well-being of students" (DASH, 2005)

- **School-site health promotion for staff**– opportunities for staff members to improve their health

© 2008 Jones and Bartlett Publishers, Inc. (www.jbpub.com)

Notes

Issues & Concerns Facing the Coordinated School Health Program - 1

- **Lack of Support for Coordinated School Health Programs**– research shows programs work; they are not in place in all schools, although the need is strong; many barriers:
  - Lack of: local administrative support, adequately prepared teachers, time in school day/year, money/funds, community/parental support for controversial topics, reinforcement by state & local policy makers
  - Policy constraints
  - Teacher priorities
  - Pressure to focus on subjects included on tests

© 2008 Jones and Bartlett Publishers, Inc. (www.jbpub.com)

Issues & Concerns Facing the Coordinated School Health Program - 2

- **Controversy regarding the school health curriculum**– based on differing values & religious teachings & on differences regarding the proper implementation of the curriculum
- **School-based health centers/school-linked health centers**– offer comprehensive health services; have met with resistance in certain communities mostly because of distribution of birth control products
- **Violence in schools**– risk factors need to be identified

© 2008 Jones and Bartlett Publishers, Inc. (www.jbpub.com)

Issues & Concerns Facing the Coordinated School Health Program - 3

Reducing Controversial School Health Curricula

- Implementing age-appropriate curricula
- Using qualified teachers & acceptable teaching methods
- Gaining parent/guardian approval
- Developing policy that allows parents/guardians to review the curriculum being taught & have the right to remove their child if they believe it is necessary
- Implementing policy to handle concerns from parents/guardians

© 2008 Jones and Bartlett Publishers, Inc. (www.jbpub.com)

Notes

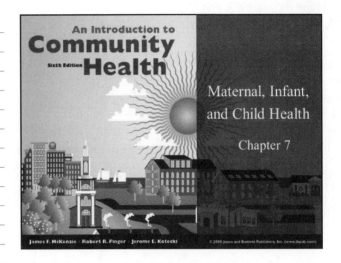

Maternal, Infant, and Child (MIC) Health

- The health of women of childbearing age from pre-pregnancy through pregnancy, labor, and delivery, the postpartum period and the health of the child prior to birth through adolescence

© 2008 Jones and Bartlett Publishers, Inc. (www.jbpub.com)

Precursors to High Rates of MIC Morbidity and Mortality

- Unintended pregnancies
- Lack of prenatal care
- Poor maternal and child nutrition
- Maternal drug use
- Low immunization rates
- Poverty
- Limited education
- Insufficient child care
- Lack of health care services in the community

© 2008 Jones and Bartlett Publishers, Inc. (www.jbpub.com)

Notes

MIC Health & Community Programs

- Many precursors/risk factors can be reduced or prevented with early intervention or educational programs or preventive medical services for women, infants, and children.
- MIC health statistics are regarded as important indicators of the effectiveness of the disease prevention and health promotion services in a community.

© Jose Luis Pelaez, Inc./Blend Images/age fotostock

© 2008 Jones and Bartlett Publishers, Inc. (www.jbpub.com)

MIC Health & Community Programs

- Early community efforts provide a positive environment that supports the physical and emotional needs of the woman, infant, and family.

- Successful efforts reduce the need for more costly medical or social assistance to these same members of society later in their lives.

© 2008 Jones and Bartlett Publishers, Inc. (www.jbpub.com)

Community Health Programs

- Have significantly reduced many of the precursors/risk factors related to MIC health over the past couple of decades

- Challenges still remain as evident by disparities among various race and ethnic groups

© 2008 Jones and Bartlett Publishers, Inc. (www.jbpub.com)

Notes

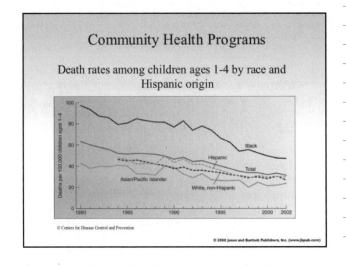

Community Health Programs

U.S Mortality Rates Among Infants Less than One Year

Black — 14.1
All races — 6.9
Hispanic — 5.9
White, non-Hispanic — 5.8

© Centers for Disease Control and Prevention

© 2008 Jones and Bartlett Publishers, Inc. (www.jbpub.com)

Community Health Programs

African American Women and White Women Who Died of Pregnancy Complications, U.S 1973-2000

No Decline
African American
White, non-Hispanic

© Centers for Disease Control and Prevention

© 2008 Jones and Bartlett Publishers, Inc. (www.jbpub.com)

Community Health Programs

Death rates among children ages 1-4 by race and Hispanic origin

Black
Hispanic
Total
Asian/Pacific Islander
White, non-Hispanic

© Centers for Disease Control and Prevention

© 2008 Jones and Bartlett Publishers, Inc. (www.jbpub.com)

Community Health Programs

Death rates among children ages 5-14 by race & Hispanic Origin

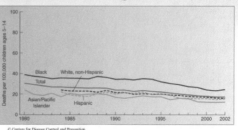

© Centers for Disease Control and Prevention

© 2008 Jones and Bartlett Publishers, Inc. (www.jbpub.com)

Family and Reproductive Health

- The family is one of society's most treasured foundations.
- Families represent a primary social group that influences and is influenced by other people and establishments.
- Families are the primary unit in which infants and children are nurtured and supported regarding their healthy development.

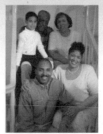

© Liquid Library

© 2008 Jones and Bartlett Publishers, Inc. (www.jbpub.com)

Family Definitions

- "A group of two people or more (one of whom is the householder) related by birth, marriage, or adoption and residing together; all such people (including subfamily members) are considered as members of one family." – *U.S. Census Bureau*

- "Two or more persons who are joined together by bonds of sharing and emotional closeness and who identify themselves as being part of a family." – *Friedman*

© 2008 Jones and Bartlett Publishers, Inc. (www.jbpub.com)

Research on the Family

- Increased health risks for infants and children who are raised in single-parent families including:
  - Adverse birth outcomes
  - Low birth weights
  - Increase in infant mortality
  - Increase of children living in poverty

© 2008 Jones and Bartlett Publishers, Inc. (www.jbpub.com)

Research on the Family

- Unmarried mothers (compared to married mothers) are more likely to have:
  - Lower education
  - Lower incomes
  - Greater dependence on welfare

- In 2004, the percentage of live births to unmarried mothers was 35.8%, or nearly double that of the 18.4% of live births to unmarried women that occurred in 1980.

© 2008 Jones and Bartlett Publishers, Inc. (www.jbpub.com)

Research on the Family

Percentage of All Births to Unmarried Women, by Age

© Data from Martin, J. A., et al. (2005). Births: Final Data for 2003. National Vital Statistics Reports 54(2): 1–30.

© 2008 Jones and Bartlett Publishers, Inc. (www.jbpub.com)

Teenage Births

- Teenagers who become pregnant and have a child are more likely than their peers who are not mothers to:
  - Drop out of school
  - Not get married or have a marriage end in divorce
  - Rely on public assistance
  - Live in poverty

Teenage Births

- Have substantial economic consequences for society in the form of increased welfare costs
  - $7 billion annually in direct costs associated with health care, foster care, and public assistance

- Result in serious health consequences for these women and their babies
  - Less likely to receive prenatal care

Teenage Births

Characteristics of teenage mothers and mothers, U.S, 1999

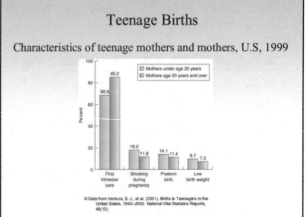

Data from Ventura, S. J., et al. (2001). Births to Teenagers in the United States, 1940–2000. National Vital Statistics Reports, 49(10).

Effective Community Health Programs

- Due in large part to effective community health programs and public health campaigns aimed at reducing teenage pregnancies, teen pregnancy, and birth rates have steadily declined in recent years.
  - Between 1991 and 2004, the teenage birth rate in the U.S. declined 33% to a record low of 41.2 births per 1,000 teenage girls in 2004.
  - Despite the recently declining rates, 31% of teenage girls get pregnant once before they reach age 20, resulting in approximately 750,000 pregnancies a year.

© 2008 Jones and Bartlett Publishers, Inc. (www.jbpub.com)

Family Planning

- Defined as the process of determining the preferred number and spacing of children in one's family and choosing the appropriate means to achieve this preference

- Effective family planning includes preconception education, good gynecological, maternal, and child care

© 2008 Jones and Bartlett Publishers, Inc. (www.jbpub.com)

Family Planning

BOX 7.2 — TEN GREAT PUBLIC HEALTH ACHIEVEMENTS, 1900–1999: FAMILY PLANNING

Changes in Family Planning

In 1900, the average life span was 47 years, and 10% of infants died during their first year of life. The average woman had 3.5 children, and 6 to 9 women per 1,000 died in childbirth. Distribution of information regarding contraception and contraceptive devices was generally illegal under federal and state Comstock laws, which had been enacted in the late 1800s. In 1900, the most common methods of contraception included withdrawal before ejaculation, rhythm, contraceptive douches, and vaginal pessaries (diaphragms, for example).

Milestones in Family Planning, United States, 1900–1999

1914	Margaret Sanger arrested for distributing information regarding birth control
1916	First birth control clinic, Brooklyn, New York, closed after 10 days by the New York City Vice Squad
1917	Federal registration of birth certificates
1928	Timing of ovulation during the menstrual cycle established
1955	First national fertility survey
1960	First licensure of birth control pills
1960	Modern intrauterine device licensed
1965	*Griswold v. Connecticut*; Supreme Court legalizes contraception
1970	Title X created
1972	Medicaid funding for family planning services authorized
1972	*Roe v. Wade*; Supreme Court legalizes abortion
1973	First National Survey of Family Growth taken
1990	Norplant licensed
1992	Depo-Provera licensed
1993	Female condom licensed

Source: Available at http://www.cdc.gov/pllen/tema/achievements/family2/fp2.htm

© 2008 Jones and Bartlett Publishers, Inc. (www.jbpub.com)

Notes

Family Planning

- Governmental health programs
  - Title X of Public Health Service Act
  - Medicaid
  - Maternal and Child Health Bureau
  - Social Service Block Grants
  - State funds

© 2008 Jones and Bartlett Publishers, Inc. (www.jbpub.com)

Family Planning Clinics

- Title X provides funding support to approximately 61% of the 4,000-plus family planning clinics nationwide
  - Annually, 4.8 million women receive health care services at family planning clinics funded by Title X
  - Serve predominantly young, poor, uninsured, and have never had a child

© 2008 Jones and Bartlett Publishers, Inc. (www.jbpub.com)

Family Planning Clinics

Family planning agencies offer a range of services beyond contraception.

	0	10	20	30	40	50	60	70	80	90	100
Nutrition counseling											
Immunizations											
Postpartum care											
Well-baby care											
WIC program											
Prenatal care											
Sports/work physicals											
Infertility counseling											
Primary health care											
Midlife health											
Colposcopy											

% of publicly supported agencies

© Alan Guttmacher Institute (2000). *Fulfilling the Promise: Public Policy and U.S. Family Planning Clinics.* New York: Author, 18. Reprinted with permission.

© 2008 Jones and Bartlett Publishers, Inc. (www.jbpub.com)

Abortion

- *Roe v. Wade*
  - A 1973 Supreme Court decision that made it unconstitutional for state laws to prohibit abortions

- As a result of Roe v. Wade, the number of women dying from illegal abortions has diminished sharply during the last 3 decades in the U.S.

Abortion

Number, ratio, and rate of abortions performed each year, U.S

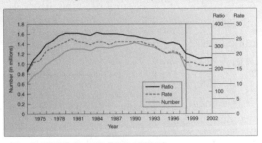

© Strauss, L.T., et al. (2005). Morbidity and Mortality Weekly Report, 54(SS 7): 1–15.

Pro-life vs Pro-choice

- Pro-life
  - A medical/ethical position that holds that performing an abortion is an act of murder

- Pro-choice
  - A medical /ethical position that holds that women have a right to reproductive freedom

Maternal Health & Mortality

- Maternal health: The health of women in the childbearing years, including those in the pre-pregnancy period, those who are pregnant, and those who are caring for young children

- Maternal mortality: The death of a woman while pregnant or within 42 days of termination of pregnancy, irrespective of the duration and site of the pregnancy, from any cause related to or aggravated by the pregnancy or its management but not from accidental or incidental causes

© 2008 Jones and Bartlett Publishers, Inc. (www.jbpub.com)

Prenatal Health Care

- Medical care provided to a pregnant woman from the time of conception until the birth process occurs
- It includes:
  - Risk assessment
  - Education
  - Treatment for medical conditions or risk reduction

© 2008 Jones and Bartlett Publishers, Inc. (www.jbpub.com)

Prenatal Health Care

Mothers, beginning in their First Trimester, by Race, Ethnicity

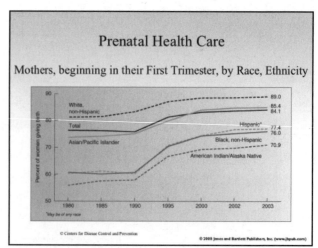

© Centers for Disease Control and Prevention

© 2008 Jones and Bartlett Publishers, Inc. (www.jbpub.com)

Infant Health Depends on

- Mother's health and her health behavior
- Mother's level of prenatal care
- Mother's quality of delivery
- Infant's environment after birth
- Proper nutrition
- Essential medical services (including postnatal physical examination by a *neonatologist*, regular visits to a physician, and the appropriate immunizations

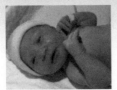

© Courtesy of Elizabeth Platt

© 2008 Jones and Bartlett Publishers, Inc. (www.jbpub.com)

Infant Mortality

- Is the death of a child younger than 1 year

- Infant death is an important measure of a nation's health because it is associated with a variety of factors including:
  - Maternal health
  - Quality of access to medical care
  - Socioeconomic conditions
  - Public health practices

© 2008 Jones and Bartlett Publishers, Inc. (www.jbpub.com)

Infant Mortality

Important Early Life Infant Mortality Periods

© Objectives for Healthy People 2000, Washington, D.C.

© 2008 Jones and Bartlett Publishers, Inc. (www.jbpub.com)

Notes

Infant Mortality

- Leading Causes
  - Congenital abnormalities
  - Preterm/low birth weight
  - Sudden infant death syndrome (SIDS)
  - Problems related to complications of pregnancy
  - Respiratory distress syndrome

© 2008 Jones and Bartlett Publishers, Inc. (www.jbpub.com)

Improving Infant Health

- Reducing premature births, which are babies born prior to 37 weeks' gestation
- Reducing low birth weight, which are infants that weigh 5.5 pounds or less at birth
- Reducing smoking during pregnancy
- Eliminating heavy maternal alcohol use
- Increasing breastfeeding rates
- Placing babies on their back to sleep

© 2008 Jones and Bartlett Publishers, Inc. (www.jbpub.com)

Child Health (ages 1-14)

- Is essential to each child's optimal development

- Failure to provide timely and remedial care leads to unnecessary illness, disability, and death – events that are associated with much greater costs than the timely care itself

© 2008 Jones and Bartlett Publishers, Inc. (www.jbpub.com)

Child Health (ages 1-14)

Leading Causes of Death in Children, 1-14

Ages 1-4

Cause	Rate
Unintentional injury	10.6
Congenital malformations	3.3
Malignant neoplasms	2.4
Homicide	2.2
Diseases of the heart	1.2
Influenza and pneumonia	1.0
Septicemia	0.05

Ages 5-14

Cause	Rate
Unintentional injury	6.3
Malignant neoplasms	2.6
Congenital malformations	0.9
Homicide	0.8
Suicide	0.6
Diseases of the heart	0.6
Influenza and pneumonia	0.3

Death rate per 100,000 population in specified age group

© National Center for Health Statistics

© 2008 Jones and Bartlett Publishers, Inc. (www.jbpub.com)

Childhood Morbidity

- Unintentional injuries

- Maltreatment

- Infectious diseases

© 2008 Jones and Bartlett Publishers, Inc. (www.jbpub.com)

Community Programs

- Over 35 health programs in 16 different agencies serve the needs of our nation's children.

- Maternal and Child Health Bureau
  - Maternal and Child Health Service Block Grant Program
  - The Healthy Start Initiative
  - Emergency Medical Services for Children Program
  - The Abstinence Education Program

© 2008 Jones and Bartlett Publishers, Inc. (www.jbpub.com)

Women, Infants, and Children (WIC) Program

- A clinic-based program designed to provide a variety of nutritional and health-related goods and services to pregnant, postpartum, and breastfeeding women, infants, and children under age 5
- Program criteria
  - Reside in the state in which applying
  - Meet the income guidelines
  - Are determined to be at "nutritional risk" by a health care professional

© 2008 Jones and Bartlett Publishers, Inc. (www.jbpub.com)

Women, Infants, and Children Program

Trends in WIC Program Participation, 1977-2004

© USDA. Used with permission.

© 2008 Jones and Bartlett Publishers, Inc. (www.jbpub.com)

Government Health Insurance for Women, Infants, and Children

- Medicaid
  - Health care program for low-income children
  - Early and periodic screening, diagnostic, and treatment program

- State Children's Health Insurance Program
  - Targets low-incomes families that do not qualify for Medicaid

© 2008 Jones and Bartlett Publishers, Inc. (www.jbpub.com)

Government Health Insurance for Women, Infants, and Children

Percentage of Children Covered by Health Insurance

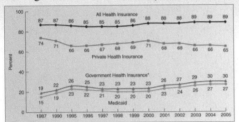

© Child Trends Data Bank

© 2008 Jones and Bartlett Publishers, Inc. (www.jbpub.com)

Providing Child Care

- Family and Medical Leave Act (FMLA)
  - Grants 12 weeks of unpaid leave to men or women after the birth of a child, an adoption, or in the event of illness in the immediate family

- Family Support Act
  - Provides funding for child care assistance to welfare parents who are employed or participating in an approved training program

© 2008 Jones and Bartlett Publishers, Inc. (www.jbpub.com)

Other Advocates for Children

- Children's Defense Fund (CDF)

- United Nations Children's Fund

- American Academy of Pediatrics

© 2008 Jones and Bartlett Publishers, Inc. (www.jbpub.com)

Notes

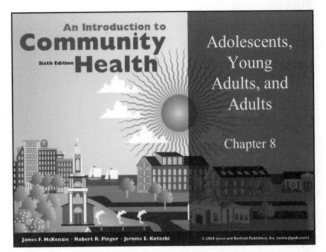

Introduction

- **Adolescents & young adults: 15–24 yrs. of age**
- **Adults: 25–64 yrs. of age**
- **15-64 yrs. most productive years of life (complete formal education, raise families, select career, etc.)**
- **Understanding age group health risks & problems:**
  - Detect risks for specific priority populations
  - Propose specific risk reduction programs

© 2008 Jones and Bartlett Publishers, Inc. (www.jbpub.com)

Adolescents & Young Adults - 1

- **15-24 yrs. old; very important because they are the future**

- **Two subgroups**
  - Puberty to maturity– face hormonal changes, physical maturation, & frequent opportunities to engage in risky behavior
  - Young adults– face many physical, emotional, & educational changes (e.g., completion of physical development & maturity, marriages, starting families & careers)

© 2008 Jones and Bartlett Publishers, Inc. (www.jbpub.com)

Adolescents & Young Adults - 2

- **This stage in life can be the most difficult due to:**
  - Increased freedom
  - Access to health-compromising substances & experiences
  - Lifestyle challenges
- **A critical stage in developing good health beliefs, attitudes, & behavior**

©SW Productions/Jupiterimages

© 2008 Jones and Bartlett Publishers, Inc. (www.jbpub.com)

Adolescents & Young Adults - 3
Demography

- **Number of Adolescents and Young Adults–** Peaked at 21% in 1979 with baby boomers; in 2005 the number was just over 14%; ~66% were white
- **Living Arrangements–** In 2005, 32% lived in single-parent homes; 66% of black children lived in single-parent homes
- **Employment Status–** has remained relatively constant since 1980

© 2008 Jones and Bartlett Publishers, Inc. (www.jbpub.com)

Adolescents & Young Adults - 4
Labor force participation by young adults

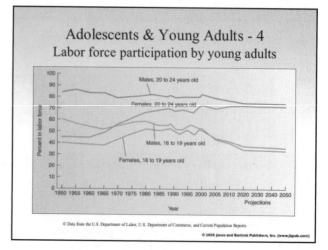

© Data from the U.S. Department of Labor, U.S. Department of Commerce, and Current Population Reports

© 2008 Jones and Bartlett Publishers, Inc. (www.jbpub.com)

Adolescents & Young Adults - 5
Health Profile

- **Mortality**
  - Death rate declined
  - Threat comes primarily from behavioral activities
  - Higher rates in men
- **Causes**
  - Unintentional injuries (mostly from vehicle crashes); many include use of alcohol
  - Homicides; up from 1950
  - Suicides; up from 1950; higher in males

© 2008 Jones and Bartlett Publishers, Inc. (www.jbpub.com)

Adolescents & Young Adults - 6
Death Rates

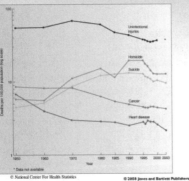

© National Center For Health Statistics

© 2008 Jones and Bartlett Publishers, Inc. (www.jbpub.com)

Adolescents & Young Adults - 7
Health Profile

- **Morbidity**
  - Communicable diseases: measles, STDs (most prevalent– chlamydia, gonorrhea)
  - Almost half of STD infections in U.S. each year occur in this age group
  - Several STDs can be treated but not cured, e.g., hepatitis, HIV, HPV
  - Age group most likely to have multiple sex partners & engage in unprotected sex

© 2008 Jones and Bartlett Publishers, Inc. (www.jbpub.com)

Adolescents & Young Adults - 8
Health Profile

- **Health behaviors & lifestyle choices for H.S. students**
  - Unintentional injuries: lack of seat belt & helmet use, use of alcohol

  - Violence: carrying weapons, fighting, rape, suicide

  - Tobacco use: ~ 1/4 smoke; ~ 1/12 use smokeless tobacco; both are down from previous years

Adolescents & Young Adults - 9
Health Profile

- **Health behaviors & lifestyle choices for H.S. students (continued)**
  - Alcohol & other drugs: alcohol & marijuana
  - Sexual behavior that leads to unintended pregnancy & STDs: ~ 50% engaged in sexual intercourse; 750,000 pregnancies each year, which is down
  - Physical activity: ~1/3 inactive; females more so
  - Overweight & weight control: many overweight & many have engaged in weight loss behaviors

Adolescents & Young Adults - 10
Health Profile

- **Health behaviors & lifestyle choices for college students**
  - Unintentional injuries: motor vehicle crashes– lack of seat belt; driving, boating, or swimming while using alcohol; riding with others who drink & drive
  - Violence: sexual assault
  - Tobacco use: ~ 1/4 smoke, similar to U.S. population

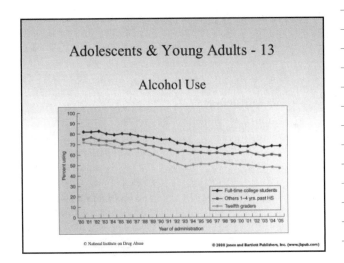

Notes

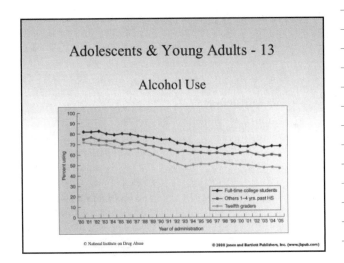

Slide: Adolescents & Young Adults - 11 — Cigarette Use

Slide: Adolescents & Young Adults - 12 — Health Profile

- **Health behaviors & lifestyle choices for college students (continued)**
  - Alcohol & other drugs: ~ 68% drink; ~1/5 use illicit drugs

  - Sexual behavior that leads to unintended pregnancy & STDs: condom use low

© 2008 Jones and Bartlett Publishers, Inc. (www.jbpub.com)

Slide: Adolescents & Young Adults - 13 — Alcohol Use

Notes

Adolescents & Young Adults - 14
Strategies for Improving Health

- **Social & cultural factors are important**

- **Community-wide** (involving stakeholders)

- **Comprehensive**

- **Collaborative**

- **Multifaceted**

© 2008 Jones and Bartlett Publishers, Inc. (www.jbpub.com)

Adults - 1
Health Profile

- **Mortality**
  - 25-44 yrs. of age: unintentional injuries, cancer, heart disease, suicide, homicide, HIV
  - 45-64 yrs. of age: cancer, heart disease, unintentional injuries, diabetes, stroke, CLRD
- **Cancer**
  - #1 killer in this age group
  - Most prevalent types: lung, colorectal, breast
  - Screenings important to catch early

© 2008 Jones and Bartlett Publishers, Inc. (www.jbpub.com)

Adults - 2
Health Profile

- **Cardiovascular Diseases**
  - Death rates continue to drop

  - This drop has vaulted cancer to be #1 killer in 45–65-year-olds

  - Change due primarily to public health efforts aimed at decreasing smoking, increasing exercise, & eating better

© 2008 Jones and Bartlett Publishers, Inc. (www.jbpub.com)

Adults - 3
Health Behaviors & Lifestyle Choices

- **Personal action can substantially decrease risk of ill health**
- **Risk factors for chronic disease**
  - Single best behavioral change– stop smoking

  - Exercise: only 22% get enough to achieve fitness

  - Overweight & obese: ~ 2/3 of 20–74-year-olds; of these about 1/2 are overweight & 1/2 obese

© 2008 Jones and Bartlett Publishers, Inc. (www.jbpub.com)

Adults - 4

Obesity, 2005

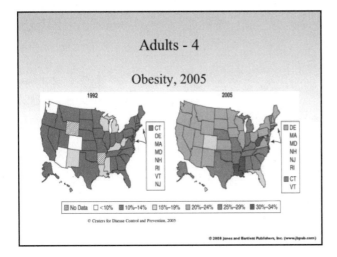

© Centers for Disease Control and Prevention, 2005

© 2008 Jones and Bartlett Publishers, Inc. (www.jbpub.com)

Adults - 5
Health Behaviors & Lifestyle Choices
(continued)

- **Risk factors for personal injury**
  - Motor vehicles: not wearing seat belts & using alcohol; both regulated by public health laws

- **Awareness & screening of certain medical conditions**
  - Noninvasive or minimally invasive health screenings for hypertension, diabetes, hypercholesterolemia & cancer

© 2008 Jones and Bartlett Publishers, Inc. (www.jbpub.com)

Adults - 6
Strategies for Improving Health

- **Primary prevention**– e.g., exercise & nutrition programs

- **Secondary prevention**– e.g., clinical screenings

- **Tertiary prevention**– e.g., medication compliance

Notes

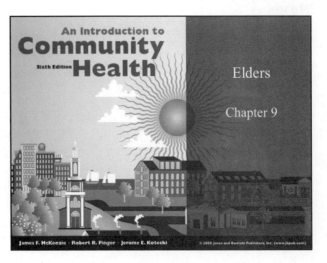

Introduction

- **American population is growing older**

- **Number of elders in America increased dramatically in the twentieth century**

- **Age is and always will be a relative concept**

© 2008 Jones and Bartlett Publishers, Inc. (www.jbpub.com)

Definitions - 1

- **Old** (≥ 65), **young old** (65-74), **middle old** (75-84), **old old** (≥ 85)
- **Aged**– state of being old
- **Aging**– changes that occur as living things grow older
- **Gerontology**– study of aging from the broadest perspective
- **Geriatrics**– medical practice specializing in treatment of the aged

© 2008 Jones and Bartlett Publishers, Inc. (www.jbpub.com)

Notes

Definitions - 2

- **Elders**– those 65 years of age and older

- **Ageism**– prejudice and discrimination against the aged

- **Elderhostel**– education programs specifically for elders held on college campuses

---

Myths Surrounding Aging - 1

- **None of these are true!**
  - "After age 65, life goes steadily downhill."
  - "Old people are all alike."
  - "Old people are lonely & ignored by their families."
  - "Old age used to be better."
  - "Old people are senile."

Myths Surrounding Aging - 2

- **None of these are true (continued)!**
  - "Old people have the good life."
  - "Most old people are sickly."
  - "Old people no longer have any sexual interest or ability."
  - "Most old people end up in nursing homes."
  - "Older people are unproductive."

Demography of Aging - 1

- **Demography**– the study of a population and those variables bringing about change in that population

- **Size & growth of the elder population**
  - In 2005, 1 in 8 $\geq$ 65
  - Baby boomers begin to turn 65 in 2011.
  - In 2030, 71 million people (1 in 5) will be $\geq$ 65
  - Old old is the fastest-growing population
  - In 2035, median age will peak at 38.7

© 2008 Jones and Bartlett Publishers, Inc. (www.jbpub.com)

Demography of Aging - 2

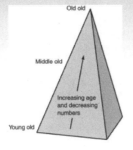

© 2008 Jones and Bartlett Publishers, Inc. (www.jbpub.com)

Demography of Aging - 3

- **Factors that affect population size & age**
  - Fertility rates: number of births per 1000 women ages 15-44

  - Mortality rate: deaths per 100,000 population; steady last 20+ years; interacts with life expectancy

  - Migration and net migration: movement from one country to another; highest after Civil War

© 2008 Jones and Bartlett Publishers, Inc. (www.jbpub.com)

Demography of Aging - 4

- **Dependency and labor-force ratios**
  - Dependency ratio: comparison of economically unproductive and economically productive

  - Total dependency ratio: comparison of both youth and elderly to economically productive

  - Youth dependency ratio: comparison of youth to economically productive

© 2008 Jones and Bartlett Publishers, Inc. (www.jbpub.com)

Demography of Aging - 5

- **Dependency and labor-force ratios (continued)**
  - Elderly dependency ratio: comparison of elderly to economically productive

  - Labor-force ratio: comparison of workers to nonworkers regardless of age

  - The ratio of workers to nonworkers will be lower in the future than today

© 2008 Jones and Bartlett Publishers, Inc. (www.jbpub.com)

Demography of Aging - 6

Youth and Elderly Dependency Rates

© Data from the U.S Bureau of the Census and Current Population Records.

© 2008 Jones and Bartlett Publishers, Inc. (www.jbpub.com)

Demography of Aging - 7

- **Other demographic variables: Marital status**
  - More elder men are married than women because they (1) have shorter life expectancies, (2) tend to marry women younger than themselves, (3) are more likely to remarry if they lose their spouse—thus, most men have spouse assistance
  - Number of divorced elders will continue to rise; causing financial troubles for many
  - Single elders with social networks get along fine

© 2008 Jones and Bartlett Publishers, Inc. (www.jbpub.com)

Demography of Aging - 8

- **Other demographic variables: living arrangements**
  - Older people who live alone are more likely to live in poverty than elders who don't
  - 2/3 of elderly live with someone
  - 4% of elderly live in nursing homes; most are women; over 1/2 over 85 years old
  - Percent in nursing homes down because of assisted living facilities

© 2008 Jones and Bartlett Publishers, Inc. (www.jbpub.com)

Demography of Aging - 9

- **Other demographic variables: race & ethnicity**
  - In 2004, most (82%) are white but that will change in years ahead

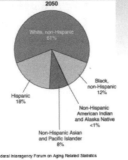

© Federal Interagency Forum on Aging Related Statistics

© 2008 Jones and Bartlett Publishers, Inc. (www.jbpub.com)

Notes

_____

_____

_____

_____

_____

_____

_____

_____

_____

_____

_____

_____

_____

_____

_____

_____

_____

_____

_____

_____

_____

_____

_____

_____

_____

_____

_____

_____

Demography of Aging - 10

- **Other demographic variables: geographic distribution**
  - Just over 1/2 live in 10 states: CA, FL, IL, MI, NJ, NY, NC, OH, PA, TX
  - CA has the most
  - FL has greatest percentage
  - Several Midwest states have small total number but high percentage

Demography of Aging - 11

- **Other demographic variables: economic status**
  - In 1970, 25% of elderly lived in poverty, in 2004 it was 10%
  - Income sources

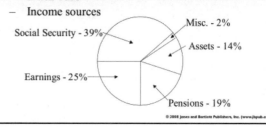

Social Security - 39%
Misc. - 2%
Assets - 14%
Earnings - 25%
Pensions - 19%

Demography of Aging - 12

- **Other demographic variables: housing**
  - Most live in adequate, affordable housing
  - But homes are older, lower value, greater need of repair, less likely to have central heating and AC, and telephones

Mobile homes - 6%

Multiunit structures - 20%

Single family homes - 75%

Health Profile of Elders - 1

- **Mortality**
  - In 2004, leading causes of death were heart disease, cancer, stroke, CLRD, and Alzheimer's disease

  - Age-adjusted death rate continues to fall

  - Biggest increase in death rates has been in diabetes & CLRD

© 2008 Jones and Bartlett Publishers, Inc. (www.jbpub.com)

Health Profile of Elders - 2

- **Morbidity**
  - Chronic conditions– hypertension, arthritis, heart disease, diabetes, emphysema; substantial burden on health & economics; 34% of elders limited by a chronic condition

  - Impairments– deficit in function of one's sense organs or limitations in one's mobility or range of motion; four primary impairments: hearing, orthopedic, cataracts, & other visual

© 2008 Jones and Bartlett Publishers, Inc. (www.jbpub.com)

Health Profile of Elders - 3

- **Health behaviors & lifestyle choices**
  - Report better health behaviors than younger people
  - Less likely to: (1) consume large amounts of alcohol, (2) smoke cigarettes, (3) be overweight & obese
  - Most important: diet, exercise & immunizations
  - Physical activity decreases with age; only 22.4% report regular physical activity

© 2008 Jones and Bartlett Publishers, Inc. (www.jbpub.com)

Notes

Notes

Health Profile of Elders - 4

- **Elder abuse & neglect**
  - Females are abused at a higher rate than men
  - Elders $\geq$ 80 years are abused or neglected at 2-3 times the rate of their proportion of the elderly
  - In 90% of abuse cases the perpetrator is a family member, and 2/3 of the perpetrators are adult children or spouses
  - Victims of self-neglect are usually depressed, confused, or extremely frail
  - Elders are frail, vulnerable, unable to defend

© 2008 Jones and Bartlett Publishers, Inc. (www.jbpub.com)

Instrumental Needs of Elders - 1

- **6 instrumental needs determine lifestyles of people of all ages: income, housing, personal care, health care, transportation, and community facilities and services**

- **Not much lifestyle change in young old**

- **More lifestyle change in middle old & old old**

© 2008 Jones and Bartlett Publishers, Inc. (www.jbpub.com)

Instrumental Needs of Elders - 2

- **Income**
  - Needs reduced in elderly
  - Increased expenses in health care & home maintenance
  - Average Social Security payment in 2006 was $1,044/month
  - Nonmarried women & minorities highest percentage in poverty

© 2008 Jones and Bartlett Publishers, Inc. (www.jbpub.com)

Instrumental Needs of Elders - 3

- **Housing**
  - 4 major needs: appropriateness, accessibility, adequacy, and affordability
  - Need housing with accommodations
  - Moving housing is difficult
  - Nursing home cost $64,000+

© 2008 Jones and Bartlett Publishers, Inc. (www.jbpub.com)

Instrumental Needs of Elders - 4

- **Housing (continued)**
  - New alternatives: Eden Alternative; Green Houses
  - Others: retirement communities; continuing-care retirement communities (CCRCs)
  - Assisted living residence

© 2008 Jones and Bartlett Publishers, Inc. (www.jbpub.com)

Instrumental Needs of Elders - 5

- **Personal Care**
  - 4 different levels of tasks: instrumental tasks (e.g., housekeeping), expressive tasks (e.g., emotional support), cognitive tasks, (e.g., scheduling appointments), and tasks of daily living (e.g., bathing)
  - Activities of daily living (ADLs) (i.e., tasks of daily living): used to define functional limitations
  - Instrumental activities of daily living (IADLs): measure more complex tasks (e.g., preparing meals)

© 2008 Jones and Bartlett Publishers, Inc. (www.jbpub.com)

Notes

Instrumental Needs of Elders - 6

- **Personal Care (continued)**
  - Informal caregiver: unpaid caregiver
  - Care provider: determines need and performs caregiving
  - Care manger: helps to determine need, but does not provide the care
  - Many problems with caregiving: money, freedom, privacy

Instrumental Needs of Elders - 7

- **Health Care**
  - Elders are the heaviest users; doctors' visits and hospital stays
  - Medicare covers much of the care; 4 parts— A, B, C, D; D the newest—prescription coverage
  - *Medigap*– fills coverage gaps of Medicare

Instrumental Needs of Elders - 8

- **Transportation**
  - Of prime importance to remain independent
  - Three different groups: those who use available transportation, those who use public transportation when there are no barriers, those who need special services
  - Solutions to transportation problems: (1) fare reductions, (2) subsidies to mass transit to reduce barriers, (3) subsidies for taxi fares, (4) funds to assist centers in purchasing equipped vehicles

Notes

Instrumental Needs of Elders - 9

- **Community Facilities & Services**
  - Older American Act of 1965 (OAA): nutrition program, State & Area Agencies on Aging, caregiver program
  - Meal service: Meals on Wheels & congregate meals
  - Homemaker service: enables elderly to remain in their own homes
  - Chore & home maintenance service
  - Visitor service for homebound

Instrumental Needs of Elders - 10

- **Community Facilities & Services (continued)**
  - Adult day care: provides care for seniors left alone all day
  - Respite care to allow caregivers some "time off"
  - Home health care: helps elders to continue to live at home
  - Senior centers: multipurpose facilities
  - Other services: specific to communities

Notes

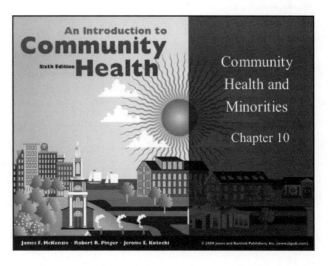

Overview of Diversity

- As America rapidly becomes the world's first truly multiracial democracy, race relations remains an issue that too often divides the nation and keeps the American dream from becoming a reality for all Americans.

- President's Initiative on Race (1997)
  - Goal was to strengthen our shared foundation as Americans so we can all live in an atmosphere of trust and understanding

© 2008 Jones and Bartlett Publishers, Inc. (www.jbpub.com)

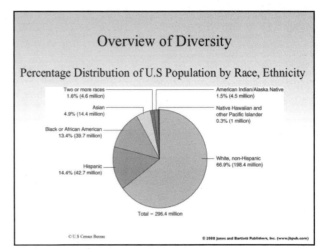

Overview of Diversity

Percentage Distribution of U.S Population by Race, Ethnicity

Two or more races
1.6% (4.6 million)

Asian
4.9% (14.4 million)

Black or African American
13.4% (39.7 million)

Hispanic
14.4% (42.7 million)

American Indian/Alaska Native
1.5% (4.5 million)

Native Hawaiian and other Pacific Islander
0.3% (1 million)

White, non-Hispanic
66.9% (198.4 million)

Total = 296.4 million

© U.S Census Bureau

© 2008 Jones and Bartlett Publishers, Inc. (www.jbpub.com)

Overview of Diversity

Projected U.S Population by Race and Hispanic Origin

© U.S Census Bureau

© 2008 Jones and Bartlett Publishers, Inc. (www.jbpub.com)

Diversity and Health

- "Advances in medical technology, lifestyle improvements, and environmental protections have all led to health gains. Yet these changes have not produced equal benefit in some racial and ethnic populations. This is the continuing challenge to public health professionals and the standard we must keep in mind when measuring our progress: what is the health status of the least empowered among us?"
Centers for Disease Control and Prevention 1997.

© 2008 Jones and Bartlett Publishers, Inc. (www.jbpub.com)

Landmark 1985 Report

- *The Secretary's Task Force Report on Black and Minority Health* (1985)
  - First documented the health status disparities of minority groups in the United States
  - Contributed significantly to the *Healthy People 2000* Objectives (1990)

© 2008 Jones and Bartlett Publishers, Inc. (www.jbpub.com)

Race and Health Initiative

- *Initiative to Eliminate Racial and Ethnic Disparities in Health* (1998)
  - Purpose was to enhance efforts in:
  - (1) Preventing Disease
  - (2) Promoting Health
  - (3) Delivering care to racial and ethnic communities

© 2008 Jones and Bartlett Publishers, Inc. (www.jbpub.com)

Racial and Ethnic Classifications

- U.S. Office of Management and Budget
  - Directive 15 "Race and Ethnic Standards for Federal Statistics and Administrative Reporting" presents brief rules for classifying into 4 racial and 2 ethnic categories. (1978)

- Revised standards issued in 1997 and expanded race from 4 to 5 categories.

© 2008 Jones and Bartlett Publishers, Inc. (www.jbpub.com)

Race and Ethnic Classifications

- Race
  - American Indian or Alaskan Native
  - Asian
  - Pacific Islander
  - Black
  - White
- Ethnicity
  - Hispanic origin or not of Hispanic origin

© 2008 Jones and Bartlett Publishers, Inc. (www.jbpub.com)

Notes

Race and Ethnic Classifications

FIGURE 10.4
U.S. Census 2000 form questions for race and ethnicity.

© 2008 Jones and Bartlett Publishers, Inc. (www.jbpub.com)

Health Data Sources and Their Limitations

- Gaps in the information system

- Bias analysis

- Self-reported data

- Reliability

© 2008 Jones and Bartlett Publishers, Inc. (www.jbpub.com)

Americans of Hispanic Origin

- Americans of Hispanic Origin
  - In 2005, 42.7 million or 14.4% of U.S. population
  - Largest minority group in America
  - Lowest education levels
  - Lower incomes
  - Higher poverty rates
- Religious beliefs play important role in health
  - Good health is seen as a matter of fortune or reward from God for good behavior.

© 2008 Jones and Bartlett Publishers, Inc. (www.jbpub.com)

Black Americans

- Black Americans
  - Having origins in any of the black racial groups from Africa
  - In 2005, 39.7 million or 12.3% of U.S. population
  - Second largest minority group in America
  - Lower education levels
  - Lowest incomes
  - Higher poverty rates
- Traditional health beliefs
  - Include curing illnesses w/ roots, herbs, barks, and teas.

© 2008 Jones and Bartlett Publishers, Inc. (www.jbpub.com)

Asian Americans

- Asian Americans
  - Refers to people of Asian descent. They or their ancestors came from more than 20 different Asian countries.
  - In 2005, 14.4 million or 4.9% of U.S. population
  - Higher education levels
  - Higher incomes
  - Lower poverty rates
- Traditional health beliefs
  - Concept of balance is related to health, and imbalance is related to disease.

© 2008 Jones and Bartlett Publishers, Inc. (www.jbpub.com)

Pacific Islander

- Pacific Islander
  - Includes peoples of Hawaii, Guam, Samoa, or other Pacific Islands and their descendants
  - In 2005, nearly 1 million or 0.3% of U.S. population
  - Lower education levels
  - Lower incomes
  - Higher poverty rates
- Traditional health beliefs
  - Healer cannot be reimbursed directly for his or her therapeutic work.

© 2008 Jones and Bartlett Publishers, Inc. (www.jbpub.com)

Notes

Notes

American Indian and Alaska Natives

- American Indian and Alaska Natives
  - Original inhabitants of America
  - In 2005, nearly 4.5 million or 1.5% of U.S. population
  - Lower education levels
  - Lower incomes
  - Higher poverty rates
- Traditional health beliefs
  - Strive for a close integration within the family, clan, and tribe and live in harmony with their environment.

Indian Health Service (IHS)

- Four goals for success:
  - Assist Indian tribes in developing health programs
  - Facilitate and assist Indian tribes in coordinating health resources
  - Provide comprehensive health care services
  - Serve as a Federal advocate

Indian Health Service

Indian Health Service Structure

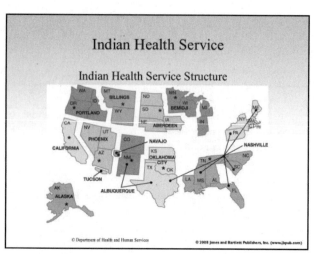

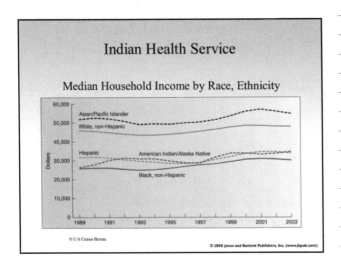

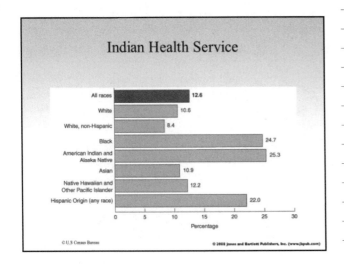

Notes

Refugees: The New Immigrants

- Refugees: People who flee their homes from danger.
- Immigrants: Migrate from other countries to set up residence in another country.
- Aliens: People who were not born in a particular country.
- Illegal aliens: Entered a country without permission.
- Special concerns
  - Poor
  - Lower levels of education
  - Few work skills
  - Serious health problems

© 2008 Jones and Bartlett Publishers, Inc. (www.jbpub.com)

Race and Health Initiative

- Infant mortality
- Cancer screening and management
- Cardiovascular diseases
- Diabetes
- HIV Infection/AIDS
- Adult and child immunizations

© 2008 Jones and Bartlett Publishers, Inc. (www.jbpub.com)

Race and Health Initiative

Infant Mortality Rates by Race, Hispanic Origin of the Mother

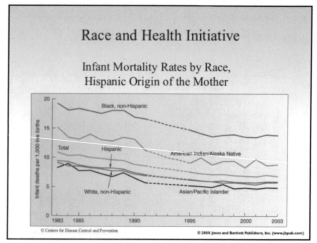

© Centers for Disease Control and Prevention

© 2008 Jones and Bartlett Publishers, Inc. (www.jbpub.com)

Race and Health Initiative

Percentage of Infants with Low Birth Weights, by Mother's Race, Hispanic Origin

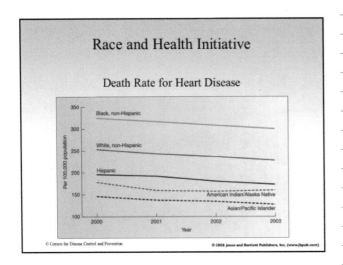

© Centers for Disease Control and Prevention   © 2008 Jones and Bartlett Publishers, Inc. (www.jbpub.com)

Race and Health Initiative

Death Rate for Heart Disease

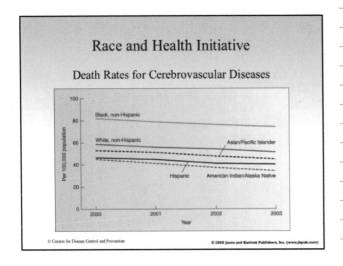

© Centers for Disease Control and Prevention   © 2008 Jones and Bartlett Publishers, Inc. (www.jbpub.com)

Race and Health Initiative

Death Rates for Cerebrovascular Diseases

© Centers for Disease Control and Prevention   © 2008 Jones and Bartlett Publishers, Inc. (www.jbpub.com)

Notes

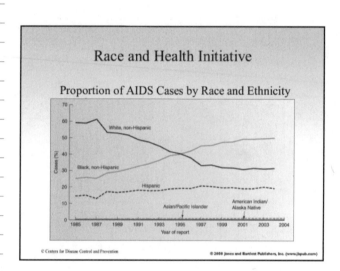

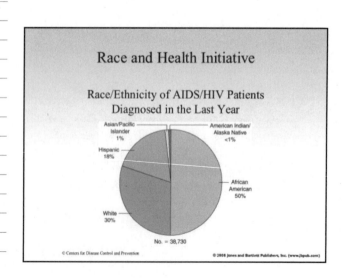

Race and Health Initiative

Vaccination Coverage by Race

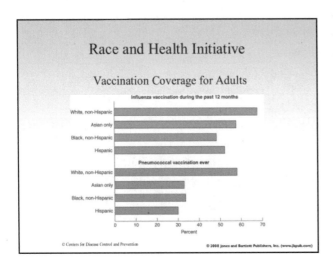

© Centers for Disease Control and Prevention

© 2008 Jones and Bartlett Publishers, Inc. (www.jbpub.com)

Race and Health Initiative

Vaccination Coverage for Adults

Influenza vaccination during the past 12 months

- White, non-Hispanic
- Asian only
- Black, non-Hispanic
- Hispanic

Pneumococcal vaccination ever

- White, non-Hispanic
- Asian only
- Black, non-Hispanic
- Hispanic

Percent

© Centers for Disease Control and Prevention

© 2008 Jones and Bartlett Publishers, Inc. (www.jbpub.com)

Socioeconomic Status & Racial and Ethnic Disparities in Health

- Socioeconomic status
  - Relating to a combination of social and economic factors
  - Has been considered the most influential single contributing factor to premature morbidity and mortality

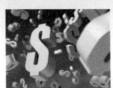

© Jong Kiam Soon/Shutterstock, Inc.

© 2008 Jones and Bartlett Publishers, Inc. (www.jbpub.com)

Notes

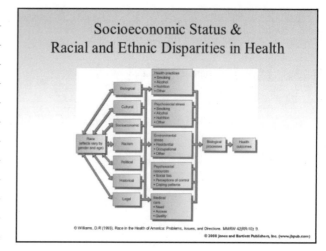

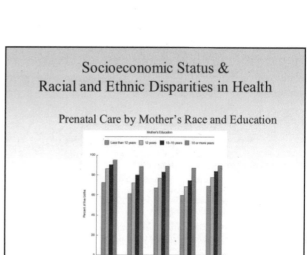

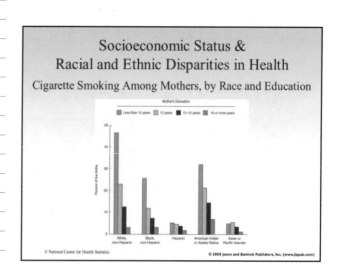

Community Health Strategies for Achieving Equity in Minority Health

- Cultural & Linguistic Competence
  - A set of congruent behaviors, attitudes, and policies that come together in a system, agency, or among professionals that enables effective work in cross-cultural situations
- Ten principles related to cultural competence
  - Considered important when planning and implementing health promotion/disease prevention programs

© 2008 Jones and Bartlett Publishers, Inc. (www.jbpub.com)

Ten Principles Related to Cultural Competence

1. Have a self understanding of race, ethnicity, and power
2. Understand historical factors
3. Understand psycho-social stressors
4. Understand cultural differences within minority groups
5. Understand minority client within the family life cycle and in an intergenerational conceptual framework

© 2008 Jones and Bartlett Publishers, Inc. (www.jbpub.com)

Ten Principles Related to Cultural Competencies

6. Understand the differences between culturally acceptable behaviors of psychopathological characteristics
7. Understand indigenous healing practices
8. Understand cultural beliefs of health
9. Understand health service resources for minority patients
10. Understand public health policies

© 2008 Jones and Bartlett Publishers, Inc. (www.jbpub.com)

Notes

_____

Community Health Strategies for
Achieving Equity in Minority Health

- Empowering the Self and the Community
  - Social power
  - Political power
  - Psychological power

Chapter 11: Community Mental Health

Notes

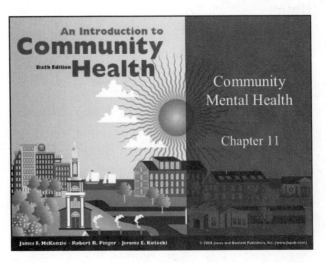

Introduction - 1

- **Mental illness: leading cause of disability in U.S., Canada, & Western Europe**
- **Mental illness is a major community health issue**
  - 22–23% (44 million) of American adults affected
  - 6% have addictive behaviors
  - 3% have both mental & addictive disorders
  - Only 1/4 to 1/3 of those diagnosed receive treatment
  - 5 million adults in U.S. have serious mental illness

© 2008 Jones and Bartlett Publishers, Inc. (www.jbpub.com)

Introduction - 2

- **Number of those affected continues to rise and affects all ages**

- **Significant resources are required to meet the continuing demands for care**

© 2008 Jones and Bartlett Publishers, Inc. (www.jbpub.com)

Notes

Key Definitions - 1

- **Mental health**– "state of successful performance of mental function, resulting in productive activities, fulfilling relationships with other people, and the ability to adapt to change and to cope with adversity" (HHS, 1999).
- **People with good mental health are able to:** function under adversity, change or adapt to changes around them, maintain control over their tension and anxiety, find more satisfaction in giving than receiving, show consideration for others, curb hate and guilt, and love others

© 2008 Jones and Bartlett Publishers, Inc. (www.jbpub.com)

Key Definitions - 2

- **Mental illness**– "a term that refers collectively to all diagnosable mental disorders" (HHS, 1999)

- **Mental disorders**– "health conditions characterized by alterations in thinking, mood, or behavior (or some combinations thereof) associated with distress and/or impaired functioning" (HHS, 1999).

- **Classification**
  - *Diagnostic & Statistical Manual of Mental Disorders,* 4th edition, text revision (*DSM-IV-TR*)
  - Classify: onset age; severity (mild, moderate, severe)

© 2008 Jones and Bartlett Publishers, Inc. (www.jbpub.com)

Origins & Causes of Mental Disorders

- **Origin:** hereditary, environmental, or both; idiopathic (unknown origin)
- **Causes:** deficiency at birth (genetic, idiopathic, maternal exposure), physical impairment, psychological
- **2/3 of mental retardation cases traceable to environmental factors** (i.e., no prenatal care, poor nutrition, DAT, postnatal exposure)

© 2008 Jones and Bartlett Publishers, Inc. (www.jbpub.com)

Notes

Mental Illness In America - 1

- **Mental illness one of the most pervasive public health problems in U.S.**
- **Statistical indicators**
  - 15.4% of adults have had at least 1 incident of a mental health or substance abuse disorder in the past 30 days
  - About 35% of the population aged 15 to 54 have had a mental disorder in their lifetime
  - Many mental disorders are chronic

© 2008 Jones and Bartlett Publishers, Inc. (www.jbpub.com)

Mental Illness in America - 2

- **Social indicators**
  - 30,000 suicides each year
  - Homicides are the 2nd & suicides are the 3rd leading cause of death in the 15-24 year olds
  - High rate of divorce
  - Current widespread abuse DAT

© 2008 Jones and Bartlett Publishers, Inc. (www.jbpub.com)

Mental Illness in America - 3

- **Stress: Contemporary mental health problem**
  - One's psychological & physiological response to stressors (stimuli in physical & social environment)
  - Selye's General Adaptation Syndrome (GAS): alarm reaction, resistance, exhaustion
  - Fight or flight reaction
  - Diseases of adaptation: e.g., ulcers, hypertension, CAD

© 2008 Jones and Bartlett Publishers, Inc. (www.jbpub.com)

Mental Illness in America - 4

- **Stress (continued)**
  - Stress impacts health via physiological or behavioral changes
  - Relationship between stress & mental health is complicated
  - Avoiding stressful situations is better than managing stress
  - Stress management is more a personal than community health matter

© 2008 Jones and Bartlett Publishers, Inc. (www.jbpub.com)

History of Mental Care in America - 1

- **Mental Health Care before WWII**
  - Colonial America: family responsibility
  - 18th century: institutions for the insane; treatment was harsh
  - Moral Treatment Era: more humane; removed from everyday stressors
  - Dorothea Dix (1802-97): advocate for those with mental illness; felt state was responsible
  - Number of state hospitals grew rapidly during last 25 years of 19th century

© 2008 Jones and Bartlett Publishers, Inc. (www.jbpub.com)

History of Mental Care in America - 2

- **Mental Health Care before WWII (continued)**
  - Mental Hygiene Movement (1st decades of 20th century)
  - Dr. Adolf Meyer (1866–1950): felt acute care should be provided in new psychopathic hospitals
  - Clifford Beers (1876–1943): bipolar mood disorder; was repeatedly hospitalized; founded what is now called the National Mental Health Association
  - By 1940, care in crowded mental hospitals became subsistence care

© 2008 Jones and Bartlett Publishers, Inc. (www.jbpub.com)

History of Mental Care in America - 3

- **Mental Health Care before WWII (continued)**
  - In 1940s new treatments: electroconvulsive therapy (ECT) & lobotomy
  - ECT: electric current used to produce convulsions; introduced in U.S. in 1939 & was popular until 1960s
  - Lobotomy: severance of nerve fibers in the brain; between 1939 & 1951, 18,000 conducted in U.S.
  - 1950s introduction of antipsychotic & antidepressive drugs

© 2008 Jones and Bartlett Publishers, Inc. (www.jbpub.com)

History of Mental Care in America - 4

- **Mental Health Care after WWII**
  - WWII conscientious objectors (COs) founded the National Mental Health Foundation & served in mental health agencies & publicized deterioration of mental hospitals
  - *National Mental Health Act of of 1946*: established National Institute of Mental Health
  - In early 1950s, people began to realize the plight of the state mental hospitals

© 2008 Jones and Bartlett Publishers, Inc. (www.jbpub.com)

History of Mental Care in America - 5

- **Mental Health Care after WWII**
  - Deinstitutionalization: discharging of patients from state-owned mental hospitals to less restrictive community settings
  - Deinstitutionalization: began in 1950s and continued through 1980s
  - Deinstitutionalization propelled by– economics, idealism, legal considerations, & antipsychotic drugs

© 2008 Jones and Bartlett Publishers, Inc. (www.jbpub.com)

History of Mental Care in America - 6

- **Mental Health Care after WWII**
  - 1961: report of the Joint Commission on Mental Illness & Health (JCMIH): recommended acute mental illness be treated in community-based settings
  - 1963: President Kennedy was concerned & the *Mental Retardation Facilities & Community Mental Health Centers (CMHC) Act* was passed
  - 1966 to 1989: 750 community mental health centers created & eligible for Medicare dollars if core services provided
  - Transinstitutionalized costs shifted to federal level

© 2008 Jones and Bartlett Publishers, Inc. (www.jbpub.com)

History of Mental Care in America - 7

- **Mental Health Care after WWII**
  - 1970s & 1980: recognition of the failure of CMHCs to meet the needs of the deinstitutionalized mentally ill
  - Initiation of Community Support Program (CSP) to promote recovery in persons with serious & persistent mental disorders
  - CSPs recognized chronic mental illness problems as social welfare problems
  - CSPs focus on service not facilities

© 2008 Jones and Bartlett Publishers, Inc. (www.jbpub.com)

Mental Health Care Concerns in America Today - 1

- **America still does not have a national mental health program**
- **Serious Mental Illness in People Who are Homeless**
  - 637,000 people are homeless in any given week in U.S.
  - 2/3 of all people with serious mental illness have been homeless
  - High prevalence of mental health, alcohol, & drug problems in homeless

© 2008 Jones and Bartlett Publishers, Inc. (www.jbpub.com)

Mental Health Care Concerns in America Today - 2

- **New asylums: Mental Care in Jails & Prisons**
  - More than 1/2 of inmates have mental health problems

Table 11.3
Prevalence of Mental Health Problems among Inmates in American Prisons and Jails, 2005

Mental Health Problem	State Prison Inmates		Federal Prison Inmates		Local Jail Inmates	
	Number	Percentage	Number	Percentage	Number	Percentage
Any mental health problem*	705,600	56.2	70,200	44.8	479,900	64.2
No mental health problem	549,000	43.8	86,500	55.2	267,600	35.8
Estimated number of inmates (June 30, 2005)	1,255,514	100.0	156,643	100.0	747,529	100.0

*Details do not add to totals because of rounding.

Source: Table developed from data provided in: James, D. J., and L. E. Glaze (2006). *Mental Health Problems of Prison and Jail Inmates.* Bureau of Justice Statistics Special Report (NCJ pub. no. 213600). Available at www.ojp.usdoj.gov/bjs/pub/.

© 2008 Jones and Bartlett Publishers, Inc. (www.jbpub.com)

Mental Health Care Concerns in America Today - 3

- **Others at high risk for mental illness** (post-traumatic stress disorder [PTSD] & major depression)
  - Citizens exposed to disasters

  - Soldiers returning from combat: ~20%

© 2008 Jones and Bartlett Publishers, Inc. (www.jbpub.com)

Meeting the Needs of those with Mental Illness - 1

- **Prevention**
  - Primary prevention: Efforts aimed at forestalling the onset of mental illness

  - Secondary prevention: Reducing the prevalence by shortening episodes

  - Tertiary prevention: Treatment & rehabilitation to ameliorate the illness & prevent further problems for the individual & the community

© 2008 Jones and Bartlett Publishers, Inc. (www.jbpub.com)

Notes

Meeting the Needs of those with Mental Illness - 2

- **Preventive Services**
  - Primary prevention: Falls on voluntary agencies like the National Mental Health Association

  - Secondary prevention: Provided by private clinics, CMHCs, ERs, & various social service providers

  - Tertiary prevention: Two basic treatment approaches– psychotherapy & psychopharmacology

© 2008 Jones and Bartlett Publishers, Inc. (www.jbpub.com)

Meeting the Needs of those with Mental Illness - 3

- **Treatment Approaches**
  - Goals: reduce symptoms, improve personal & social functioning, develop & strengthen coping skills, & promote behaviors that improve life
  - Psychotherapy: treatment through verbal communication; types–supportive, psychodynamic, & cognitive-behavioral therapy
  - Psychopharmacology: treatment with medications
  - Self-help support groups: groups united through shared interest, concern, or deficit (e.g., AA)

© 2008 Jones and Bartlett Publishers, Inc. (www.jbpub.com)

Meeting the Needs of those with Mental Illness - 4

- **Federal Initiatives for Mental Health Care**
  - Money for research, surveillance, & goal setting, little for prevention, early intervention & treatment
  - 1999 Surgeon General's Report put mental health problems "front & center"
  - 2002, President Bush formed the New Freedom Commission on Mental Health: Commission has identified major issues & a vision for a "transformed system" of mental health care but provides no road map

© 2008 Jones and Bartlett Publishers, Inc. (www.jbpub.com)

Meeting the Needs of those with Mental Illness - 5

- **Federal Initiatives for Mental Health Care (continued)**
  - Federal agencies that deal with mental health issues: HHS, National Institute of Mental Health (NIMH), & the Substance Abuse and Mental Health Services Administration (SAMHSA)
  - SAMSHA: The Center for Substance Abuse Treatment (CSAT), The Center for Substance Abuse Prevention (CSAP), Center for Mental Health Services (CMHS)

© 2008 Jones and Bartlett Publishers, Inc. (www.jbpub.com)

Meeting the Needs of those with Mental Illness - 6

- **Community Mental Health & Managed Care**
  - Cost containment
  - Behavioral health care services: only care that is "medically necessary"
  - Managed behavioral health care organizations (MBHOs): special MCOs to deal with mental health issues
  - Movement toward using only evidence-based practices

© 2008 Jones and Bartlett Publishers, Inc. (www.jbpub.com)

Meeting the Needs of those with Mental Illness - 7

- **Community Mental Health & Managed Care (continued)**
  - Parity: refers to treating the financing of mental health on the same basis of general health care
  - 1996 Mental Health Parity Act: fell short of complete parity
  - Today still not full parity in health care coverage between general health care services & mental (behavioral) health care services

© 2008 Jones and Bartlett Publishers, Inc. (www.jbpub.com)

Chapter 12: Alcohol, Tobacco, And Other Drugs: A Community Concern

Notes

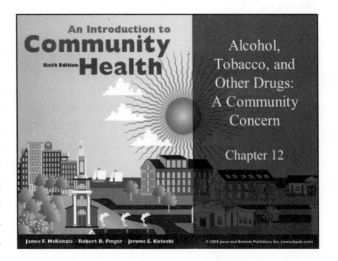

Introduction

- **Use, misuse & abuse of mind-altering substances predates recorded history**
- **Reasons for drug use**
  - Experimental or social
  - Temporary departure from natural non-drug state
  - Misguided attempt to self-medicate
  - Cope with personal problems
  - Drug dependent
- **Most cultures see abusive behavior as destructive**

© 2008 Jones and Bartlett Publishers, Inc. (www.jbpub.com)

Scope of Current Drug Problem in the U.S. - 1

- #1 community health problem in U.S.
- Substance abuse $414–$487 billion annual economic loss

Drug	Estimated Deaths	Costs (billions)
Alcohol	100,000	$220
Tobacco	430,000	$157
Illicit drugs	16,000	$110
Total	546,000	$487

© 2008 Jones and Bartlett Publishers, Inc. (www.jbpub.com)

Notes

Violence Associated with the Use of Alcohol and Other Drugs

Alcohol and other drugs are associated with

- Up to 50% Spousal abuse
- 20-35% Suicides
- 50% Traffic fatalities
- 62% Assaults
- 49% Murders
- 52% Rapes
- 68% Manslaughter charges
- 38% Child abuse
- 69% Drownings

© National Clearinghouse for Alcohol and Drug Information (1995). *Making the [Fact sheets]. Rockville, MD: Author.

© 2008 Jones and Bartlett Publishers, Inc. (www.jbpub.com)

Scope of Current Drug Problem in the U.S. - 3

- **From *Monitoring the Future* surveys**
  - Use up from 15 years ago

  - Marijuana use: 19.8% of H.S. seniors in 2005, compared to 22.4% in 2001, & 11.9% in 1992

  - Illicit drug use: 10.3% of H.S. seniors in 2005, compared to 11% in 2001, & 6.3% in 1992

  - Personal & community consequences

© 2008 Jones and Bartlett Publishers, Inc. (www.jbpub.com)

Key Definitions - 1

- **Drug:** Substance, other than food or vitamins that, when taken in small quantities, alters one's physical, mental, or emotional state

- **Psychoactive drugs:** those drugs that alter sensory perceptions, mood, thought processes, or behavior

- **Drug misuse:** inappropriate use of prescription or nonprescription drugs

© 2008 Jones and Bartlett Publishers, Inc. (www.jbpub.com)

Key Definitions - 2

- **Drug abuse:**
  - Taking of a drug for a non-medically approved purpose
  - Continued use of a legal drug with the knowledge that it is hazardous to one's health (e.g., cigarette smoking)
  - The use of alcohol & nicotine by those who are under age
- **Drug dependence:** when one believes that a particular drug is necessary for normal functioning

© 2008 Jones and Bartlett Publishers, Inc. (www.jbpub.com)

Factors That Contribute to Substance Abuse

- **Risk factors:** those that increase the probability of drug use
- **Protective risk factors:** those that decrease the probability of drug use
- **Risk & protective factors can be either genetic (inherited) or environmental**
- **Inherited:** Inherited alcoholism– Type I & II
- **Environmental risk factors:** personal, home & family, school & peer group factors, sociocultural aspects of one's environment

© 2008 Jones and Bartlett Publishers, Inc. (www.jbpub.com)

Types of Drugs

- **Legal** (licit): Alcohol, nicotine, nonprescription drugs, & prescription drugs

- **Illegal** (illicit): Stimulants, depressants, narcotics, hallucinogens, marijuana, & other drugs

© 2008 Jones and Bartlett Publishers, Inc. (www.jbpub.com)

Notes

Types of Legal Drugs Abused - 1

- **Alcohol:**
  - # 1 drug problem in America as measured by injury, deaths, & economic costs

  - Binge drinking ≥ 5 on a single occasion for males & ≥ 4 for females

  - 26% of underage drinkers abuse or are dependent

  - 75% of H.S. seniors have used alcohol

© 2008 Jones and Bartlett Publishers, Inc. (www.jbpub.com)

Types of Legal Drugs Abused - 2

- **Alcohol (continued):**
  - Problem drinkers: those who experience personal, interpersonal, legal or financial problems because of alcohol use
  - Alcoholism: physical dependence & loss of control
  - Cost of alcohol abuse: $220 billion
  - Blood alcohol concentration (BAC): percentage of concentration of alcohol in blood; BAC of ≥ .08% considered intoxication in most states

© 2008 Jones and Bartlett Publishers, Inc. (www.jbpub.com)

Types of Legal Drugs Abused - 3

- **Alcohol (continued):**
  - Alcohol use increases risk for many types of unintentional injuries, e.g., falls, drowning, burns
  - Alcohol contributes to intentional violence, e.g., spouse abuse, murders, assaults
  - Alcohol is #1 "rape drug"
  - Fetal alcohol spectrum disorder (FASD) results from pathological drinking; included are FAS, FAE, ARBD, ARND

© 2008 Jones and Bartlett Publishers, Inc. (www.jbpub.com)

Types of Legal Drugs Abused - 4

- **Nicotine**
  - Found in cigarettes, cigars, smokeless or "spit" tobacco & pipe tobacco
  - Synar Amendment: prohibits distribution of tobacco products to those < 18 years old
  - 23.2% of H.S. seniors smoke cigarettes daily; new low
  - Smoking accounts for 438,000 deaths each year
  - Smoking accounts for a loss of $138 billion

© 2008 Jones and Bartlett Publishers, Inc. (www.jbpub.com)

Types of Legal Drugs Abused - 5

- **Nicotine**
  - Environmental tobacco smoke (ETS) or secondhand smoke is a human class A carcinogen (same as asbestos); aggravates asthma

  - Smokeless (spit) tobacco carries many risks; 8.6% use in U.S.; habit begins in junior & high school years

© 2008 Jones and Bartlett Publishers, Inc. (www.jbpub.com)

Types of Legal Drugs Abused - 6

- **Over-the-counter (OTC) drugs**
  - Legal drugs, with the exception of alcohol & tobacco, that can be purchased without a doctor's prescription
  - Regulated by the FDA
  - Misuse examples: not following dosage directions (e.g. laxatives & appetite suppressants) & taking after expiration dates

© 2008 Jones and Bartlett Publishers, Inc. (www.jbpub.com)

Types of Legal Drugs Abused - 7

- **Prescription drugs**
  - Require a physician's (or dentist's) written instructions (prescription)
  - Also, regulated by FDA
  - More than 4,000
  - Misused in similar ways as OTC plus giving one person's prescription drug to another
  - Abuse levels much lower than for alcohol & tobacco
  - Concerns: dependence, adverse drug reactions, & creating drug-resistant pathogens

© 2008 Jones and Bartlett Publishers, Inc. (www.jbpub.com)

Controlled Substances & Illegal Drugs

- **Controlled substances**
  - Those regulated by the Comprehensive Drug Abuse Control Act of 1970
  - Schedule I drugs: those with high potential for abuse & no medical use (e.g., heroin, MDMA)
  - Schedule II to V: Have medical use & are placed in categories based on potential of abuse & risk of causing dependence
  - Drug Enforcement Administration (DEA) responsible for enforcing Comprehensive Drug Abuse Control Act

© 2008 Jones and Bartlett Publishers, Inc. (www.jbpub.com)

Types of Illegal Drugs Abused - 1

- **Marijuana** (pot)
  - Most abused illicit drug
  - Concerns: illegal, detrimental to health, brings people in contact with those involved in illegal activities, often involves polydrug use
  - 44.8% of H.S. seniors have used in lifetime
  - Resulting problems: many acute health effects (e.g., reduced concentration, slowed reaction time); chronic health conditions (e.g., damage to respiratory system & amotivational syndrome)

© 2008 Jones and Bartlett Publishers, Inc. (www.jbpub.com)

Types of Illegal Drugs Abused - 2

- **Narcotics: Opium, morphine, heroin & others**
  - Narcotics numb the senses and reduce pain; most widely abused is heroin; 1.5% of population
  - Opium poppies do not grow in U.S.
  - Produce tolerance and physical dependence
  - Affect community at several levels: crime, STD epidemics
  - Injection users are at high risk for becoming infected with bloodborne pathogens

© 2008 Jones and Bartlett Publishers, Inc. (www.jbpub.com)

Types of Illegal Drugs Abused - 3

- **Cocaine & Crack Cocaine**
  - Potent stimulant
  - 3.2% of H.S. seniors & 2 million Americans used in last 30 days
- **Hallucinogens**
  - Changes one's perceptions of the environment
  - Synesthesia: a mixing of the senses
  - Includes both naturally derived drugs (e.g., mescaline) & synthetic drugs (e.g., LSD)

© 2008 Jones and Bartlett Publishers, Inc. (www.jbpub.com)

Types of Illegal Drugs Abused - 4

- **Stimulants**
  - Increase activity of central nervous system
  - Examples include: amphetamine, methamphetamine, (called crystal, meth), crackmethcathinone (cat)
  - Tolerance builds quickly
- **Depressants**
  - Decrease activity of central nervous system; lower anxiety
  - Examples: barbiturates, benzodiazepines, methaqualone

© 2008 Jones and Bartlett Publishers, Inc. (www.jbpub.com)

Notes

Types of Illegal Drugs Abused - 5

- **Club & Designer drugs**
  - Club drugs: illicit, primarily synthetic, that are commonly found in nightclubs or raves; example: MDMA ("Ecstasy"); 5% of H.S. seniors have used MDMA; Rohypnol (flunitrazepan) known as date-rape drug
  - Designer drugs: term used to describe drugs synthesized by amateur chemists in secret labs: The Controlled Substances Analogue Act of 1986 passed to reduce flow of designer drugs

© 2008 Jones and Bartlett Publishers, Inc. (www.jbpub.com)

Types of Illegal Drugs Abused - 6

- **Anabolic drugs**
  - Protein-building drugs
  - Examples: anabolic/androgenic steroids, testosterone, & human growth hormone (HGH)
  - Shortcut to building muscle or to maturity
- **Inhalants**
  - Psychoactive, breathable chemicals
  - Used mostly by youth

© 2008 Jones and Bartlett Publishers, Inc. (www.jbpub.com)

Prevention & Control of Drug Abuse

- **Primary:** Aimed at those who have never used drugs; goal is to prevent or forestall the initiation of drug use (e.g., education, increasing costs)

- **Secondary:** Seek to reach those who have begun drug use but are not chronic drug abusers (e.g., education in schools, workplaces)

- **Tertiary:** Designed to provide drug abuse treatment and aftercare

© 2008 Jones and Bartlett Publishers, Inc. (www.jbpub.com)

Elements of Prevention - 1

- **Education**
  - Purpose of drug use education is to reduce demand for drugs
  - Examples: *Project DARE* & *Great American Smokeout*
- **Treatment**
  - Goal to remove physical, emotional, & environmental conditions that contribute to drug dependency; cost-beneficial
  - Aftercare: continuing care provided to recovering former drug abusers (e.g., AA)

© 2008 Jones and Bartlett Publishers, Inc. (www.jbpub.com)

Elements of Prevention - 2

- **Public policy**
  - Guiding principles & courses of action taken by governments to solve practical problems (e.g., drunk driving & BAC laws, taxes on alcohol)
- **Law enforcement**
  - Laws to arrest, jail, bring to trial, & sentence law breakers
  - Primary roles: control drug use, control crime related to drugs, prevent crime organizations, & protect neighborhoods

© 2008 Jones and Bartlett Publishers, Inc. (www.jbpub.com)

Governmental Drug Prevention & Control Agencies & Programs - 1

- **Federal Agencies & Programs**
  - Headed up by White House Office of National Drug Control Policy: budget $12.66 billion in 2007; three priorities– prevention, treatment & interdiction
  - HHS: gets largest amount of drug budget; addresses drug problem via health promotion– like nutrition & fitness programs

© 2008 Jones and Bartlett Publishers, Inc. (www.jbpub.com)

Governmental Drug Prevention & Control Agencies & Programs - 2

- **HHS agencies**
  - Substance Abuse & Mental Health Services Administration (SAMHSA): 3 centers

  - National Institute on Drug Abuse (NIDA): largest institution in world for drug abuse research

  - Food & Drug Administration: Safety & efficacy of legal drugs

© 2008 Jones and Bartlett Publishers, Inc. (www.jbpub.com)

Governmental Drug Prevention & Control Agencies & Programs - 3

- **Department of Justice**
  - Deals with the supply side of the drug trade

  - Also maintains prisons & prisoners

  - Subgroups within department that fight drug abuse are Drug Enforcement Administration (DEA) & Bureau of Alcohol, Tobacco, Firearms, & Explosives (ATF)

© 2008 Jones and Bartlett Publishers, Inc. (www.jbpub.com)

Governmental Drug Prevention & Control Agencies & Programs - 4

- **Department of Homeland Security (DHS)**
  - Authorized by President Bush after 9/11 attacks on U.S.
  - Number of federal agencies that fight drug problem were transferred to this department (e.g., Immigrations & Custom Enforcement)
  - Receives the 3rd largest amount of funding from the national drug control budget

© 2008 Jones and Bartlett Publishers, Inc. (www.jbpub.com)

Governmental Drug Prevention & Control Agencies & Programs - 5

- **Other federal agencies**
  - Department of Veteran Affairs: treatment of drug-related health problems of veterans

  - Department of Defense: assists foreign allies to control the production of illegal drugs

  - Department of Education (DE): programs for drug-free schools

© 2008 Jones and Bartlett Publishers, Inc. (www.jbpub.com)

Governmental Drug Prevention & Control Agencies & Programs - 6

- **State & local agencies & programs**
  - State government: each state has its own agencies & laws to deal with drug problems; sometimes state laws in conflict with federal laws
  - Local agencies & programs: include law enforcement, schools, health departments, justice system, drug task force or local coordinating councils

© 2008 Jones and Bartlett Publishers, Inc. (www.jbpub.com)

Nongovernmental Drug Prevention & Control Agencies & Programs

- **Community-based drug education:** Six key features– (1) comprehensive strategy, (2) indirect approach to drug abuse prevention, (3) goal of empowering youth, (4) participatory approach, (5) culture-sensitive orientation, & (6) highly structured activities
- **School-based drug education:** DARE, student assistance programs (SAPs), & peer counseling programs
- **Workplace-based drug education:** Employee Assistance Programs (EAPs)

© 2008 Jones and Bartlett Publishers, Inc. (www.jbpub.com)

Notes

Notes

Voluntary Health Agencies

- **Many local groups working on drug problem**

- **Example agencies:** Mothers Against Drunk Drivers, Students Against Drunk Drivers, Alcoholics Anonymous, Narcotics Anonymous, American Cancer Society

- **Need to work together**

© 2008 Jones and Bartlett Publishers, Inc. (www.jbpub.com)

Notes

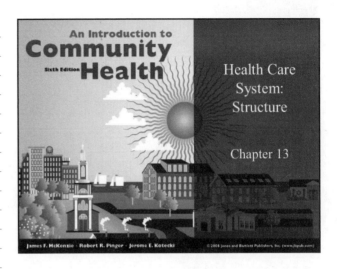

Introduction

- **Health care delivery in U.S. is different than all other developed countries**

- **Other developed countries have national health care programs run or organized by government**

- **Health care in U.S. delivered by an array of providers** (health care facilities & professionals that provide care)

© 2008 Jones and Bartlett Publishers, Inc. (www.jbpub.com)

First question…

Does the U.S. really have a
health care system?

| Providers | + | Consumers (patients) | = | System? |

© 2008 Jones and Bartlett Publishers, Inc. (www.jbpub.com)

Brief History of Health Care Delivery in the U.S. - 2

Timeline

Pre-1870   Today

© 2008 Jones and Bartlett Publishers, Inc. (www.jbpub.com)

Brief History of Health Care Delivery in the U.S. - 3

• Far behind Great Britain & Europe in both health care & medical education
• Not grounded in science
• Medical education was provided through apprenticeships

Pre-1870

© 2008 Jones and Bartlett Publishers, Inc. (www.jbpub.com)

Brief History of Health Care Delivery in the U.S. - 4

• Health care provided in patients' homes
• Hospitals in large cities & seaports
• Almshouses (poorhouse) to provide food, shelter & basic care for indigent

Pre-1870

© 2008 Jones and Bartlett Publishers, Inc. (www.jbpub.com)

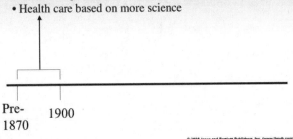

Brief History of Health Care Delivery
in the U.S. - 5

• Health care moved from patients' homes to physician's
office & hospitals
• Health care based on more science

Pre-1870   1900

© 2008 Jones and Bartlett Publishers, Inc. (www.jbpub.com)

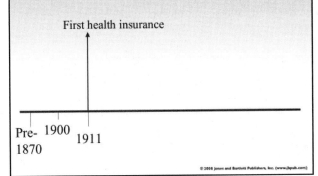

Brief History of Health Care Delivery
in the U.S. - 6

First health insurance

Pre-1870   1900   1911

© 2008 Jones and Bartlett Publishers, Inc. (www.jbpub.com)

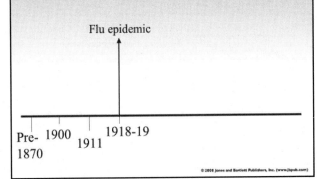

Brief History of Health Care Delivery
in the U.S. - 7

Flu epidemic

Pre-1870   1900   1911   1918-19

© 2008 Jones and Bartlett Publishers, Inc. (www.jbpub.com)

Notes

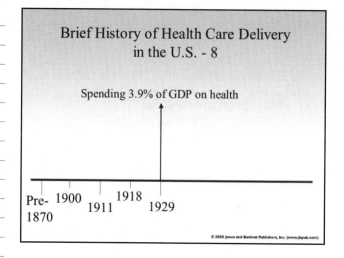

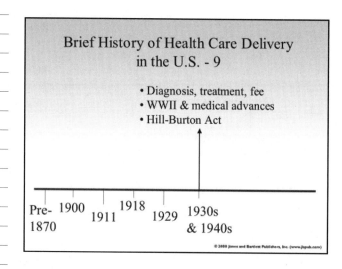

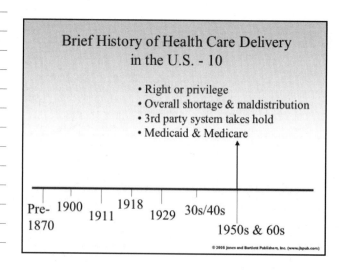

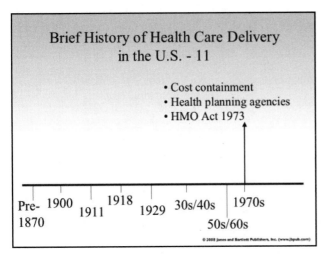

Notes

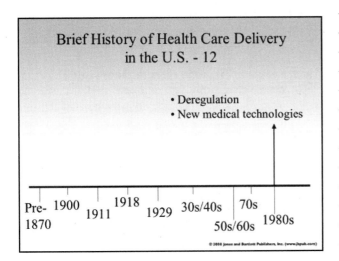

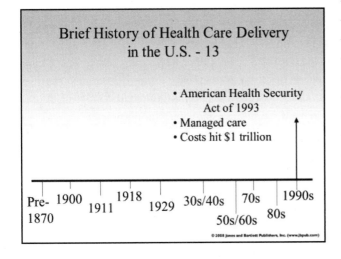

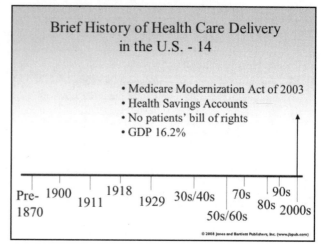

Brief History of Health Care Delivery in the U.S. - 14

- Medicare Modernization Act of 2003
- Health Savings Accounts
- No patients' bill of rights
- GDP 16.2%

Pre-1870 1900 1911 1918 1929 30s/40s 50s/60s 70s 80s 90s 2000s

© 2008 Jones and Bartlett Publishers, Inc. (www.jbpub.com)

Spectrum of Health Care Delivery - 1

- **Spectrum of care refers to the type of health care practice**
- **Population-based Public Health Practice** (health promotion & disease prevention)
- **Medical Practice**
  - Primary Care: clinical preventive services; 1st contact; front-line
  - Secondary Care: specialized attention (acute & subacute care); e.g., ERs
  - Tertiary Care: Subspecialty referral

© 2008 Jones and Bartlett Publishers, Inc. (www.jbpub.com)

Spectrum of Health Care Delivery - 2

- **Long-term practice**
  - Restorative care: intermediate follow-up
  - Long-term care: care for chronic conditions; personal care

- **End-of-life practice**
  - Care provided in last six months of life: hospice care

© 2008 Jones and Bartlett Publishers, Inc. (www.jbpub.com)

Types of Health Care Providers - 1

- **In 2005, 14 million health care workers; 9.9% of workforce**
- **42% work in hospitals as compared to 63% in 1970**
- **Over 200 different careers in the health care industry**
- **Six categories:** independent providers, limited care providers, nurses, nonphysician practitioners, allied health care professionals, public health professionals

© 2008 Jones and Bartlett Publishers, Inc. (www.jbpub.com)

Types of Health Care Providers - 2

- **Independent providers:** health care professionals with the education & legal authority to treat any health problem

- **Allopathic providers:** MDs; their remedies produce effects different from those of the disease

- **Osteopathic providers:** DOs; their remedies emphasize the interrelationships of the body's systems in diagnosis, prevention, & treatment

© 2008 Jones and Bartlett Publishers, Inc. (www.jbpub.com)

Types of Health Care Providers - 3

- **Nonallopathic providers:** independent providers who provide nontraditional forms of health care
- **Examples:** chiropractors (adjusts spinal column), acupuncturists, naturopaths, herbalists, homeopaths
- **Five general categories of complementary & alternative medicine (CAM):** Alternate medical systems, mind/body interventions, biologically-based therapy, manipulative methods, energy therapy

© 2008 Jones and Bartlett Publishers, Inc. (www.jbpub.com)

Types of Health Care Providers - 4

- **Limited care** (restricted care) **providers:** those who provide care for a specific part of the body

- **Examples**: dentists, optometrists, podiatrists, & psychologists

© 2008 Jones and Bartlett Publishers, Inc. (www.jbpub.com)

Types of Health Care Providers - 5

- **Nurses**
  - Licensed Practical (Vocational) Nurses (LPNs): 1-2 years of training & carry out nontechnical duties
  - Registered Nurses (RN): diploma or associate degree & state license
  - Professional nurses: Bachelor of Science in Nursing (BSN); prepared for additional activities involving independent judgment
  - Advanced Practice Nurses (APN): master's or doctoral degrees; e.g., nurse practitioners, clinical nurse specialists, certified nurse midwife

© 2008 Jones and Bartlett Publishers, Inc. (www.jbpub.com)

Registered Nurses Prepared for Advance Practice, 2004

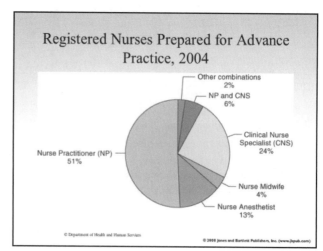

Nurse Practitioner (NP) 51%
Other combinations 2%
NP and CNS 6%
Clinical Nurse Specialist (CNS) 24%
Nurse Midwife 4%
Nurse Anesthetist 13%

© Department of Health and Human Services

© 2008 Jones and Bartlett Publishers, Inc. (www.jbpub.com)

Types of Health Care Providers - 6

- **Nonphysician Practitioners** (also known as nonphysician clinicians or midlevel providers or physician extenders

- **Examples:** nurse practitioners (NPs) & physician assistants (PAs)

© 2008 Jones and Bartlett Publishers, Inc. (www.jbpub.com)

Types of Health Care Providers - 7

- **Allied health care professionals**
  - Provide services that assist, facilitate, & complement work of physicians & other health care specialists
  - Examples: dietitians, physical therapists, medical technologists, EMTs, speech therapists, & exercise physiologists

© 2008 Jones and Bartlett Publishers, Inc. (www.jbpub.com)

Types of Health Care Providers - 8

- **Public health professionals**
  - A health care worker who works in a public health organization
  - Examples: environmental health workers, public health administrators, epidemiologists, health educators, & biostatisticians

© 2008 Jones and Bartlett Publishers, Inc. (www.jbpub.com)

Health Care Facilities & Their Accreditation - 1

- **Health care facilities:** physical settings
- **Practitioner offices:** privately owned practices
- **Clinics:** no beds; tax-supported clinics for medically indigent called public health clinics or community health centers

Health Care Facilities & Their Accreditation - 2

- **Hospital types**
  - Provide secondary & tertiary care
  - Private (proprietary or investor-owned); specialty (provide mainly one type of medicine)
  - Public (government run or funded)
  - Voluntary (not-for-profit)
  - Types of service: full-service; limited-service

Health Care Facilities & Their Accreditation - 3

- **Outpatient & ambulatory care facilities:** those that provide a wide array of outpatient services; they can range from hospital-based facilities to independently owned freestanding facilities
- Include: primary care centers, urgent/emergent care centers, ambulatory surgery centers, diagnostic imaging centers
- Some found in nontraditional settings

Health Care Facilities & Their Accreditation - 4

- **Rehabilitation Centers**
  - Used to restore lost functions
  - Ambulatory & inpatient facilities
- **Long-term Care Options**
  - Residential care (e.g., nursing home & assisted living)
  - Home health care
  - Hospice, and home care

Health Care Facilities & Their Accreditation - 5

- **Accreditation:** process by which an agency or organization evaluates & recognizes an institution as meeting certain predetermined standards
- **Agencies/Organizations**
  - Joint Commission on Accreditation of Health Care Organizations (JCAHO): 15,000 facilities
  - Centers for Medicare & Medicaid Services (CMS): grants "deeming authority"

Notes

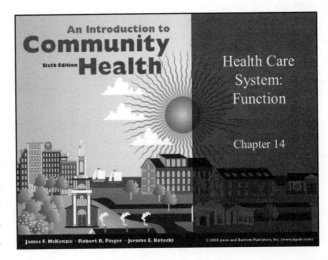

Introduction

- **This chapter includes:**
  - How consumers obtain health care services

  - How health care services are paid and who is paying the bill

  - Issues of concern: Access, quality, cost

  - Potential solutions

© 2008 Jones and Bartlett Publishers, Inc. (www.jbpub.com)

Access & Paying for Health Care

- **Health care services not accessible to all**

- **Even when accessible there are racial & ethnic disparities**

- **Major problems of system represented in Kissick's (1994) cost containment, access, & quality triangle**

© 2008 Jones and Bartlett Publishers, Inc. (www.jbpub.com)

Notes

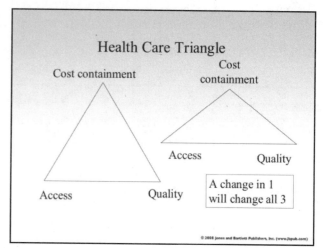

Health Care Triangle

Cost containment

Cost containment

Access

Quality

Access

Quality

A change in 1
will change all 3

© 2008 Jones and Bartlett Publishers, Inc. (www.jbpub.com)

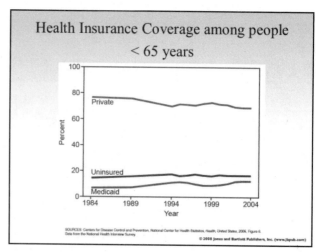

Access to Health Care - 1

- **In 2005, 46.6 million Americans were uninsured; millions more lacked coverage for shorter periods of time**
- **Likelihood of being uninsured greater for those who:** are younger, are less educated, have lower incomes, are not white, are not U.S. citizens, & are males
- **8 in 10 uninsured persons were members of working families**

© 2008 Jones and Bartlett Publishers, Inc. (www.jbpub.com)

Health Insurance Coverage among people < 65 years

SOURCES: Centers for Disease Control and Prevention, National Center for Health Statistics. Health, United States, 2006, Figure 6. Data from the National Health Interview Survey.

© 2008 Jones and Bartlett Publishers, Inc. (www.jbpub.com)

Access to Health Care - 2

- **Medically indigent:** unable to receive health care because they cannot afford health care

- **Working poor:** have a job but unable to afford health insurance; 30 million

- **Most Americans pay for health care 3 or 4 times**

© 2008 Jones and Bartlett Publishers, Inc. (www.jbpub.com)

Access to Health Care - 2

Why People Do Not Have Health Insurance?

© Adams, P. F., and P. M. Barnes (2006). Vital and Health Statistics, 10(229).

© 2008 Jones and Bartlett Publishers, Inc. (www.jbpub.com)

Quality of Health Care

- **WHO measures with disability-adjusted life expectancy (DALE)**
- **U.S. government measures with *National Healthcare Quality Report*** (effectiveness, patient safety, timeliness, & patient centeredness)
- **Accreditation**
  - JCAHO– facilities
  - National Committee on Quality Assurance– health care plans

© 2008 Jones and Bartlett Publishers, Inc. (www.jbpub.com)

Paying for Health Care - 1

- **Cost in 2006**
  - $2+ trillion
  - $7,129 per capita
  - More than any other nation
  - 16.2% of GDP; expected to reach 20% in 2015

- **4 primary sources of payment**

© 2008 Jones and Bartlett Publishers, Inc. (www.jbpub.com)

Paying for Health Care - 1

Personal Health Care Expenditure by Source of Funds

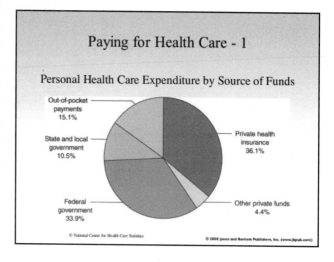

Out-of-pocket payments 15.1%

State and local government 10.5%

Federal government 33.9%

Private health insurance 36.1%

Other private funds 4.4%

© National Center for Health Care Statistics

© 2008 Jones and Bartlett Publishers, Inc. (www.jbpub.com)

Paying for Health Care - 2

- **Arrangements for payment: fee-for-service** (fee schedule) **& prepaid health care**
- **Fee-for-service:** patient (first party), provider (second party), health insurance company or government (third party)
- **Prepaid health care found mostly in managed care plans;** set price on per-member, pre-month basis– capitated fee, capitation system

© 2008 Jones and Bartlett Publishers, Inc. (www.jbpub.com)

Health Insurance - 1

- **Like other insurance– risk & cost spreading process**

- **Paid for in "equitable fashion;" some pay more if at high risk (e.g., smoking)**

- **The greater the risk the greater the premium**

- **1911: First health insurance**

© 2008 Jones and Bartlett Publishers, Inc. (www.jbpub.com)

Health Insurance - 2

- **State Children's Health Insurance Program (SCHIP)**
  - Enacted in 1997 & authorized in 1997 for $40 billion
  - To cover uninsured children: 11.3 million
  - Voluntary grants to states; can be part of Medicaid
  - In 2005, 6.1 million children were enrolled
  - Up for re-authorization in 2007

© 2008 Jones and Bartlett Publishers, Inc. (www.jbpub.com)

Health Insurance - 3

- **Health Insurance Policy:** a written agreement between an insurance company (or the government) & an individual or group of individuals to pay for certain health care costs during a certain period in return for regular, periodic payments (a set amount of money) called premiums

- **There are expectations for both sides; they are not always met**

© 2008 Jones and Bartlett Publishers, Inc. (www.jbpub.com)

Notes

Health Insurance - 4

- **Key definitions**
  - **Premiums**: regular periodic payments

  - **Deductible**: amount of money that the beneficiary must pay before the insurance company begins to pay for covered services

  - **Co-insurance**: portion of an insurance company's approved amounts for covered services that the beneficiary is responsible for paying; co-payment: type of co-insurance, a negotiated set fee

© 2008 Jones and Bartlett Publishers, Inc. (www.jbpub.com)

Health Insurance - 5

- **Key definitions (continued)**
  - **Fixed indemnity**: maximum amount an insurer will pay for a certain service
  - **Exclusion**: specific health condition that is excluded from coverage
  - **Pre-existing condition**: that which has been diagnosed or treated 6 months before health policy began; the Health Insurance Portability & Accountability Act (HIPAA) of 1996 helped to deal with this situation

© 2008 Jones and Bartlett Publishers, Inc. (www.jbpub.com)

Health Insurance - 6

- **Types of health insurance coverage**
  - **Hospitalization**: inpatient hospital expenses, including room, patient care, supplies, & medications
  - **Surgical**: surgeons' fees
  - **Regular medical**: nonsurgical service provided by health care providers; often has set amounts
  - **Long-term care**: array of supportive services

© 2008 Jones and Bartlett Publishers, Inc. (www.jbpub.com)

Health Insurance - 7

- **Types of health insurance coverage (continued)**
  - **Major medical**: large medical expenses usually not covered by regular medical or dental coverage
  - **Dental**: dental procedures
  - **Disability**: income when the insured is unable to work because of a health problem
  - **Optical**: nonsurgical procedures to improve vision

© 2008 Jones and Bartlett Publishers, Inc. (www.jbpub.com)

Health Insurance - 8

- **Though types of health insurance coverage have remained constant, several trends have emerged**
- **Trends**
  - More complex plans & concentrated in fewer companies
  - Increasing diversity of products; more options
  - Delivery of care through networks
  - Shifting financial structures & incentives
  - Managing utilization & improving quality of care

© 2008 Jones and Bartlett Publishers, Inc. (www.jbpub.com)

Health Insurance - 9

- **Cost of health insurance**
  - Cost of insurance mirrors cost of care
  - Two major factors set the cost: risk of the group, amount of coverage provided
  - 61% of employers provided health insurance in 2006; 69% in 2000
  - Employers are shifting costs to employees
  - $1,500 of the cost of each new car covers health insurance of auto makers

© 2008 Jones and Bartlett Publishers, Inc. (www.jbpub.com)

Health Insurance - 10

- **Self-insured organizations:** those that pay the health care of its employees with the premiums collected from the employees & the contributions made by the employer
  - Used to try to control cost of insurance
  - Third-party administrators usually handle the administration
  - Several benefits for organizations: set parameters, hold cash reserves, exempt from mandatory benefits law, & administrative costs grow at slower rate

© 2008 Jones and Bartlett Publishers, Inc. (www.jbpub.com)

Health Insurance Provided by the Government - 1

- **Medicare**
  - For those: (1) ≥ 65 years of age, (2) with kidney failure, & (3) certain disabilities
  - Administered by Centers for Medicare & Medicaid (CMS)
  - Paid for with employee & employer contributions; FICA tax
  - Has 4 parts: A (hospital insurance), B (medical insurance), C (managed care plans), D (prescription drugs plans)

© 2008 Jones and Bartlett Publishers, Inc. (www.jbpub.com)

Health Insurance Provided by the Government - 2

- **Medicare (continued)**
  - Part A (hospital insurance): mandatory & is provided without further cost to those eligible; can be purchased for those not eligible; has deductible & co-insurance
  - Part B (medical insurance): those with Part A are automatically enrolled unless they decline; there are income-related premiums taken directly from Social Security checks; has deductible & co-insurance

© 2008 Jones and Bartlett Publishers, Inc. (www.jbpub.com)

Health Insurance Provided by the Government - 3

- **Medicare (continued)**
  - Part C (managed care plans): called Medicare Advantage; introduced to reduce costs; includes items covered in Parts A, B, & D; often no need to purchase Medigap; not available everywhere
  - Part D (prescription drugs plans): introduced Jan. 1, 2006 as part of MMA of 2003; there are premiums; has deductible, co-insurance & "donut hole"
  - Prospective Pricing System (PPS): 470 diagnosis-related groups (DRGs) for hospital diagnosis

© 2008 Jones and Bartlett Publishers, Inc. (www.jbpub.com)

Health Insurance Provided by the Government - 4

- **Medicaid**
  - A federal-state health insurance program for the poor
  - Eligibility for programs is determined by each state; no age requirements
  - Non-contributory program
  - Very costly program for most states
  - Can be combined with the SCHIP

© 2008 Jones and Bartlett Publishers, Inc. (www.jbpub.com)

Supplemental Health Insurance - 1

- **Medigap**
  - Supplemental insurance program for Medicare
  - 12 standardized plans (A-L) defined by the federal government
  - Not needed with Medicare Advantage; Medicare *SELECT* is available in some states
- **Other supplemental insurance**
  - Disease specific
  - Fixed indemnity policies
  - Long-term care insurance; nursing home cost $64K+

© 2008 Jones and Bartlett Publishers, Inc. (www.jbpub.com)

Notes

Supplemental Health Insurance -2

- **Reasons to get long-term care insurance**
  - To preserve financial assets
  - To prevent the need for family members or friends to provide care
  - To enable people to stay independent in their homes longer
  - To make it easier to get into the nursing home or assisted living home of their choice

© 2008 Jones and Bartlett Publishers, Inc. (www.jbpub.com)

Supplemental Health Insurance - 3

Who Pays for Health Care?

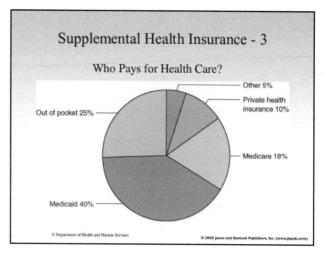

Other 5%
Private health insurance 10%
Out of pocket 25%
Medicare 18%
Medicaid 40%

© Department of Health and Human Services

© 2008 Jones and Bartlett Publishers, Inc. (www.jbpub.com)

Managed Care - 1

- **Manage health care costs by influencing patient care decisions**
- **Around since the 1970s, but took hold in 1990s**
- **In 2005, 176 million enrolled**
- **Plans managed by managed care organizations (MCOs)**

© 2008 Jones and Bartlett Publishers, Inc. (www.jbpub.com)

Managed Care - 2

- **Goals:** control costs through efficiency & coordination, reduce unnecessary or inappropriate utilization, increase access to preventive care, maintain or improve quality of care

- **Common features:** provider panels, limited choice, gatekeeping, risk sharing, quality management, & utilization review

© 2008 Jones and Bartlett Publishers, Inc. (www.jbpub.com)

Managed Care - 3

- **Types of managed care**
  - Preferred provider organizations (PPOs): closest to fee-for-service; agreement between provider & organization to provide service to members for discounted rate
  - Exclusive provider organizations (EPOs): like a PPO but with stronger financial incentives
  - Health Maintenance Organizations (HMOs): oldest form; combines insurance & medical care; uses primary care physicians & prepaid health care arrangement

© 2008 Jones and Bartlett Publishers, Inc. (www.jbpub.com)

Managed Care - 4

- **Types of HMOs**

© 2008 Jones and Bartlett Publishers, Inc. (www.jbpub.com)

Notes

Notes

Managed Care - 5

- **Types of managed care (continued)**
  - Point-of-Service Option (POS): associated with HMOs & allows for more liberal policy in selecting providers
  - Physician-Hospital Organizations (PHOs): arrangements between physicians & hospitals to negotiate with insurers as MCOs
  - Medicare Advantage: HMO option of Medicare; not available everywhere
  - Medicaid & managed care: most states use; 61% of people covered in Medicaid are in managed care

© 2008 Jones and Bartlett Publishers, Inc. (www.jbpub.com)

Managed Care - 6

- **Advantages of managed care**
  - Comprehensive benefits
  - Evidence-based high-quality care
  - Well-documented services provided through integrated delivery systems
  - Accountability for quality improvement
- **However, many Americans are still worried about health care**

© 2008 Jones and Bartlett Publishers, Inc. (www.jbpub.com)

Managed Care - 7

- **Concerns of managed care**
  - Not managed care but "managed cost"
  - Authorizing only certain practitioners under contract
  - Reviewing treatment decisions
  - Closely monitoring high-cost cases
  - Reducing inpatient stays
  - Using lower cost alternative treatments
  - Delays in receiving care
  - Cannot understand bills

© 2008 Jones and Bartlett Publishers, Inc. (www.jbpub.com)

Other Arrangements for Delivering Health Care - 1

- **National Health Insurance**
  - Implies a system in which the federal government ensures the availability of health care services for all people
  - All developed countries but one have such a system
  - Types: national health service model (e.g., U.K., Spain) & social insurance model (e.g., Canada & Germany)

© 2008 Jones and Bartlett Publishers, Inc. (www.jbpub.com)

Canadian Health Care System

- **Government - 3rd party "single payer":** fee-for-service program; select own physicians; providers accept provincial plan for reimbursement
- **Major advantages over U.S. system:** all Canadians have insurance; equity; administrative costs lower; less expensive to operate; emphasis on prevention & primary care
- **Major disadvantages -** wait lists

© 2008 Jones and Bartlett Publishers, Inc. (www.jbpub.com)

Other Arrangements for Delivering Health Care - 2

- **State plans**
  - Several states have made changes; many others in the process
  - Oregon Health Plan: revises Medicaid; addresses access first, cost second; prioritization process with list of 710; in 2006, items 1-530 were covered
  - Massachusetts Health Care Plan: began 7-1-07; mandated coverage for all paid for by employers & taxes

© 2008 Jones and Bartlett Publishers, Inc. (www.jbpub.com)

Notes

Health Care Reform in the U.S. - 1

- **6 attempts at national health insurance**
- **Reform has centered on specific portions of the system**
  – SCHIP
  – Medicare Prescription Drug Improvement and Modernization Act of 2003; Part D - prescription drug plan & health savings accounts (HSA)

Health Care Reform in the U.S. - 2

- **Health savings accounts**
  - 3 million have; give people more of a stake in spending; best for healthy & wealthy
  - How they work: Like 401(k) plans– money invested grows tax free; money withdrawn tax free to pay for care; used for anything after 65 (but must pay income tax); some employers contribute to HSA; paired with high deductible policies; have portability
  – Advantages (bring down monthly premiums) & Disadvantages (pay more out of pocket & some may skip needed care)

Health Care Reform in the U.S. - 3

- **Institute of Medicine's recommendations for reform**
  – Health care coverage should be *universal, continuous, & affordable to individuals & families.*
  – The health insurance strategy should be *affordable & sustainable for society.*
  – Health insurance should *enhance health & well-being* by promoting access to high-quality care that is effective, efficient, safe, timely, patient-centered, & equitable.

Notes

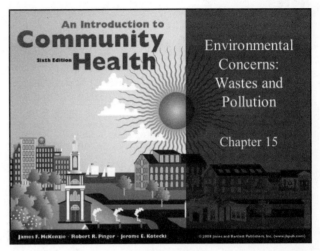

Introduction

- **Environment:** external conditions, circumstances, and influences surrounding and affecting the growth and development of an organism or a community of organisms

- **Ecology:** study of how living things interact with each other & their environment

- **Biosphere:** zone of the earth where life is found

© 2008 Jones and Bartlett Publishers, Inc. (www.jbpub.com)

Natural Environmental Hazards

- **Natural hazards:** an event of nature that increases the probability of disease, injury, or death of humans; e.g., tsunamis, floods, tornadoes, hurricanes
- **Results of natural hazards:** contaminated water & food, high temperatures, loss of shelter
- **In addition, humans can alter, pollute, & destroy their environment & thus impact health**

© 2008 Jones and Bartlett Publishers, Inc. (www.jbpub.com)

Notes

Residues & Wastes from Human Activities

- **Residues & wastes:** unwanted by-products of human activities; e.g., wastewater, garbage, trash, radioactive wastes
- **Factors contributing to environmental hazards**
  - Urbanization
  - Industrialization
  - Human population growth
  - Production & use of disposable products & containers

© 2008 Jones and Bartlett Publishers, Inc. (www.jbpub.com)

Types of Wastes & Pollution - 1

- **Disposal of wastes often pollutes natural resources** – air, land, & water
- **Solid wastes**
  - Sources: agriculture (51%), mining (38%), industry (8%), municipalities–municipal solid waste (MSW) (trash & garbage) (3%), & utilities
  - Each person produces an average of 4.5 pounds of MSW/day
  - Getting rid of it; will it decompose

© 2008 Jones and Bartlett Publishers, Inc. (www.jbpub.com)

Types of Wastes & Pollution - 2

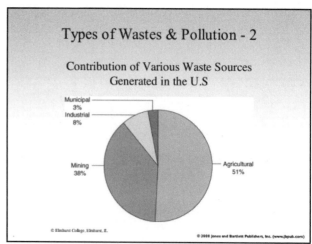

Contribution of Various Waste Sources Generated in the U.S

Types of Wastes & Pollution - 3

Types and Percentages of Solid Wastes Generated in the U.S

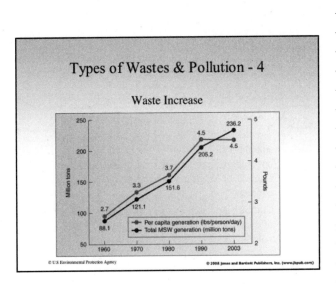

Wood 5.7%
Glass 5.2%
Rubber, leather, and textiles 7.3%
Metals 7.6%
Plastics 11.8%
Food scraps 11.9%
Other 3.4%
Paper 34.2%
Yard trimmings 13.1%

© U.S Environmental Protection Agency

© 2008 Jones and Bartlett Publishers, Inc. (www.jbpub.com)

Types of Wastes & Pollution - 4

Waste Increase

Per capita generation (lbs/person/day)
Total MSW generation (million tons)

88.1, 2.7 — 1960
121.1, 3.3 — 1970
151.6, 3.7 — 1980
205.2, 4.5 — 1990
236.2, 4.5 — 2003

© U.S Environmental Protection Agency

© 2008 Jones and Bartlett Publishers, Inc. (www.jbpub.com)

Types of Wastes & Pollution - 5

- **Solid waste management**
  - Collection: 80% of waste management money spent on this
  - Source reduction: limit creation
  - Recycling: collecting (curbside & drop-off), sorting, & processing; composting; in 2003, U.S. recycled 31% of MSW; goal is 38% by 2010

© 2008 Jones and Bartlett Publishers, Inc. (www.jbpub.com)

Notes

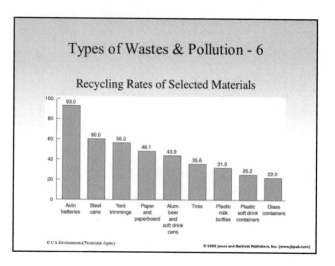

Types of Wastes & Pollution - 6

Recycling Rates of Selected Materials

Auto batteries	93.0
Steel cans	60.0
Yard trimmings	56.3
Paper and paperboard	48.1
Alum. beer and soft drink cans	43.9
Tires	35.6
Plastic milk bottles	31.9
Plastic soft drink containers	25.2
Glass containers	22.0

© U.S Environmental Protection Agency

© 2008 Jones and Bartlett Publishers, Inc. (www.jbpub.com)

Types of Wastes & Pollution - 7

- **Solid waste management** (continued)
  - **Disposal**
    - Sanitary landfills: waste disposal sites on land suited for it– waste spread in layers, compacted, & covered; primary means of disposal; RCRA (Rick-Rah) of 1976 eliminated dumps; leachates a concern
    - Combustion (incineration): Second major method of disposal (15%); reduces weight by 75% & volume by 90%; energy recovery plants

© 2008 Jones and Bartlett Publishers, Inc. (www.jbpub.com)

Types of Wastes & Pollution - 8

- **Hazardous wastes**
  - Defined: a solid waste or combination of solid wastes that is dangerous to human health & the environment
  - Defined by U.S. Environmental Protection Agency (EPA)
  - RCRA of 1976 established system of controlling from generation to disposal (*cradle-to-grave regulation*) & mandates strict controls over treatment & storage

© 2008 Jones and Bartlett Publishers, Inc. (www.jbpub.com)

Types of Wastes & Pollution - 9

- **Hazardous waste management:** 15 different methods overseen & regulated by EPA
  - Deep well injection: the pumping of liquid hazardous waste into rock lined wells below aquifers; most common means, handles 34%
  - Secured landfill & Incineration: similar principles as managing MSW but restrictions greater because of danger to health & environment; only 7% was disposed of this way
  - Source reduction: best solution; few incentives

© 2008 Jones and Bartlett Publishers, Inc. (www.jbpub.com)

Types of Wastes & Pollution - 10

- **Hazardous waste cleanup:** sites created from inappropriate disposal or abandonment
  - Big problem underground storage tanks (UST) that have leaked; concern– contamination of water & buildup of gases
  - 1980– Comprehensive Environmental Response, Compensation, and Liability Act: created priority list, makes responsible parties pay, & cleanup; called Superfund
  - Brownfields: abandoned industrial sites where cleanup & reuse are difficult

© 2008 Jones and Bartlett Publishers, Inc. (www.jbpub.com)

Air Pollution - 1

- **Air Pollution:** contamination of the air that interferes with the comfort, safety, & health of living organisms
- **Most prevalent sources of air pollution:** transportation, electric power plants, mills, & refineries
- **EPA under clean air act sets limits on pollution:** those of greatest concern are criteria air pollutants
- **National Ambient Air Quality Standards (NAAQS)**
- **Air Quality Index (AQI)**

© 2008 Jones and Bartlett Publishers, Inc. (www.jbpub.com)

Notes

Air Pollution - 2

Color Codes for Air Quality Rates

Air Quality Index Levels of Health Concern	Numerical Value	Meaning
Good (green)	0–50	Air quality is considered satisfactory, and air pollution poses little or no risk.
Moderate (yellow)	51–100	Air quality is acceptable; however, for some pollutants there may be a moderate health concern for a very small number of people who are unusually sensitive to air pollution.
Unhealthy for Sensitive Groups (orange)	101–150	Members of sensitive groups may experience health effects. The general public is not likely to be affected.
Unhealthy (red)	151–200	Everyone may begin to experience health effects; members of sensitive groups may experience more serious health effects.
Very Unhealthy (purple)	201–300	Health alert: everyone may experience more serious health effects.
Hazardous (maroon)	>300	Health warnings of emergency conditions. The entire population is more likely to be affected.

© AIRNow

© 2008 Jones and Bartlett Publishers, Inc. (www.jbpub.com)

Air Pollution - 3

- **Special Concerns with Outdoor Air**
  - Acid rain (snow, dew, drizzle, fog, & sleet): result from emissions of burning fossil fuels that react with water vapor
  - Global warming: matter of debate; caused in part by greenhouse gases, e.g., chlorofluorocarbons (CFCs), carbon dioxide, which hold in heat; small increase in temperature can affect air quality, water & health

© 2008 Jones and Bartlett Publishers, Inc. (www.jbpub.com)

Air Pollution - 4

- **Special Concerns with Outdoor Air**
  - Destruction of the ozone layer: ozone layer filters 99% of sun's harmful UV radiation; seen over polar regions; CFCs major cause of destruction
  - Photochemical smog (also called ground-level ozone): caused by combination of NO+VOC+sunlight; high percentage of Americans still exposed to high ozone levels
  - Thermal inversion: occurs when warm air traps cooler air; this traps pollutants including photochemical smog

© 2008 Jones and Bartlett Publishers, Inc. (www.jbpub.com)

Air Pollution - 5

- **Protection of Outdoor Air through Regulation**
  - Clean Air Act (CAA) of 1963: federal government authority to address interstate air pollution problems
  - 1970 amendments: First comprehensive approach to dealing with air pollution nationwide; included NAAQSs & State Implementation Plans (SIPs)
  - 1977 amendments: empowered EPA
  - 1990 amendments: to deal with urban pollution, emission controls, power plants, & ban on CFCs

© 2008 Jones and Bartlett Publishers, Inc. (www.jbpub.com)

Air Pollution - 6

- **Indoor Air**
  - Can be a greater threat to human health than outdoor air pollution
  - Air is trapped in home
  - Americans spent 80-90% of their time indoors
  - Many different sources
  - Common pollutants: asbestos, biogenic pollutants, combustion by-products, VOCs (e.g., formaldehyde, solvents, cleaners) radon, ETS (also known as 2nd hand smoke = mainstream + sidestream smoke)

© 2008 Jones and Bartlett Publishers, Inc. (www.jbpub.com)

Air Pollution - 7

- **Protection of Indoor Air**
  - 1970s energy crisis led to conservation & tight buildings
  - Sick building syndrome: air quality creates ill health
  - No standards set by federal government
  - Steps to take: select safe products, venting dryers, avoid products with formaldehyde, limit/prohibit indoor smoking, maintain heating & cooling equipment, test for radon

© 2008 Jones and Bartlett Publishers, Inc. (www.jbpub.com)

Water & Its Pollution - 1

- Clean water is needed for health & good quality of life; sanitation is also necessary
- 100% of U.S. population has clean water & sanitation
- Still U.S. has waterborne disease
- Humans & their daily activities pollute the water
- Sources of water: (1) surface (2) subsurface or groundwater (found in aquifers)

© 2008 Jones and Bartlett Publishers, Inc. (www.jbpub.com)

Water & Its Pollution - 2

- **Water pollution:** any physical or chemical change in the water that can harm living organisms or make it unfit for other uses

- **Point source pollution**: single identifiable source that discharges pollutants into the water

- **Nonpoint source pollution:** all pollution that occurs through the runoff, seepage, or falling of pollutants into the water

© 2008 Jones and Bartlett Publishers, Inc. (www.jbpub.com)

Water & Its Pollutants - 3

- **Types of water pollutants**
  - Biological pollutants: pathogens (e.g., bacteria, viruses) from runoff, failed septic tanks
  - Chemical pollutants: inorganic chemicals (e.g., lead, copper), organic chemicals (e.g., industrial solvents, pesticides, & herbicides), radioactive materials
  - Water quality in U.S. has deteriorated because of population growth, increase in chemical manufacturing, reckless land-use, disposal of hazardous wastes

© 2008 Jones and Bartlett Publishers, Inc. (www.jbpub.com)

Water & Its Pollution - 4

- **Strategies to ensure safe water**
  - Water use in U.S.: Power plants (48%), agriculture (36%), public & domestic use, & industry & mining (6%)

  - Treatment of water for use: coagulation & flocculation, sedimentation, filtration, disinfection

  - Quality of drinking water supplied by municipalities is regulated by EPA

© 2008 Jones and Bartlett Publishers, Inc. (www.jbpub.com)

Water & Its Pollution - 5

- **Wastewater treatment**
  - Wastewater: substance that remains after humans have used it for domestic & commercial purposes; includes 99.9% water & 0.1% suspended & dissolved solids
  - Purpose: to improve quality to be able to release back into environment
  - Stages of municipal water treatment: preliminary (remove large solids), primary (sedimentation that forms sludge), secondary (biological & physical treatment), tertiary (advanced; filtration)

© 2008 Jones and Bartlett Publishers, Inc. (www.jbpub.com)

Water & Its Pollution - 6

- **Wastewater treatment (continued)**
  - Septic system: watertight tank (sedimentation) & absorption field; must be located in appropriate soil, properly constructed & inspected, & maintained regularly

© 2008 Jones and Bartlett Publishers, Inc. (www.jbpub.com)

Notes

_____

_____

_____

_____

_____

_____

_____

_____

_____

_____

_____

_____

_____

_____

_____

_____

_____

_____

_____

_____

_____

_____

_____

_____

_____

_____

_____

_____

_____

_____

_____

_____

_____

_____

_____

_____

_____

_____

_____

_____

Water & Its Pollution - 7

- **Protection of water quality through regulation**
  - Surface & drinking water regulated through 2 different regulations
  - Surface water (i.e., rivers, lakes) regulated by Federal Water Pollution Control Act Amendments of 1972 & 1977– known as Clean Water Act (CWA): early efforts to control point source pollution: since 1982 more nonpoint pollution– watershed
  - Safe Drinking Water Act (SDWA): EPA sets national limits for contaminants; some would like to see this strengthened

© 2008 Jones and Bartlett Publishers, Inc. (www.jbpub.com)

Radiation - 1

- **Radiation Defined:** energy released when atoms split
- **Large doses harmful to living organisms**
- **Sources of radiation**
  - Natural: cosmic radiation (sun & outer space), terrestrial radiation (earth's minerals), & internal radiation (inside the body from ingestion)
  - Human-made: x-rays, nuclear medicine, consumer products (e.g., TVs), nuclear power plants, nuclear weapons

© 2008 Jones and Bartlett Publishers, Inc. (www.jbpub.com)

Radiation - 2

Sources of Ionizing Radiation

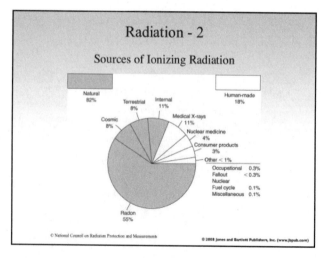

© National Council on Radiation Protection and Measurements

© 2008 Jones and Bartlett Publishers, Inc. (www.jbpub.com)

Radiation - 3

- **Nuclear power plants**
  - 103 nuclear power plants in the U.S. in 31 states

  - 20 years since a serious accident

  - Deposal of nuclear waste is a problem in U.S. (underground site in Nevada has been debated for many years), thus new nuclear power plants in U.S. are unlikely until this is resolved

© 2008 Jones and Bartlett Publishers, Inc. (www.jbpub.com)

Noise Pollution

- **Noise pollution defined:** excessive sound; unwanted sound
- **Amplitude:** sound volume measured in decibels (dB)
- **Approaches to noise abatement:** A local problem; difficult to control
  - Policy: Noise Control Act of 1972— covers new products & quiet communities
  - Educational programs: to alter behavior
  - Environmental changes: at source, during travels, to exposed parties

© 2008 Jones and Bartlett Publishers, Inc. (www.jbpub.com)

Notes

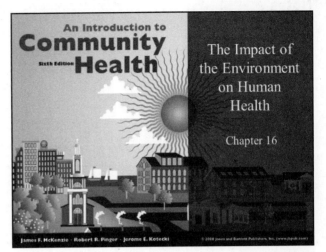

Introduction - 1

- **Environmental health defined:** study & management of environmental conditions that affect health & well-being of humans

- **Environmental hazards defined:** factors or conditions in the environment that increase the risk of human injury, disease, or death

- **All environment-induced disease is highly preventable**

© 2008 Jones and Bartlett Publishers, Inc. (www.jbpub.com)

Introduction - 2

- **Communities can limit their exposure to environmental hazards by**
  - Supporting & using recycling
  - Protecting quality of local water
  - Avoiding accumulation of trash
  - Supporting local wastewater facilities & treatment of stormwater
  - Adopting environmental sound practices for disposal of solid & hazardous waste
  - Supporting sustainable development

© 2008 Jones and Bartlett Publishers, Inc. (www.jbpub.com)

Biological Hazards & Human Health - 1

- **Biological hazards**: living organisms (& viruses), or their products, that increase the risk of disease of death in humans

- **Environmental sanitation:** the practice of establishing & maintaining healthy & hygienic conditions in the environment

- **The mismanagement of wastewater or solid waste can result in epidemic of waterborne, foodborne, & vectorborne diseases**

© 2008 Jones and Bartlett Publishers, Inc. (www.jbpub.com)

Biological Hazards & Human Health - 2

- **Waterborne diseases:** occur when contaminated water with a disease agent is consumed by a susceptible person, e.g., typhoid & cholera which have killed thousands
- **Waterborne disease outbreak (WBDO):** an event in which at least 2 persons experience a similar illness after ingestion of or exposure to water that is the probable cause of the illness; can also be caused by excessive levels of fluoride, copper & nitrates
- **Prevention:** appropriate plumbing, wastewater treatment, fluoridation (big boost to dental problems)

© 2008 Jones and Bartlett Publishers, Inc. (www.jbpub.com)

Biological Hazards & Human Health - 3

- **Foodborne diseases:** occur when contaminated food with a disease agent is consumed by a susceptible person, e.g., *salmonella, E. coli*
- **Foodborne disease outbreak (FBDO):** the occurrence of 2 or more cases of a similar illness resulting from the ingestion of food
- **Causes of FBDOs:** improper holding temperatures & inadequate cooking of food; also, poor hygiene of food preparers, contaminated equipment, & getting food from an unsafe source (e.g., seafood from polluted waters)

© 2008 Jones and Bartlett Publishers, Inc. (www.jbpub.com)

Biological Hazards & Human Health - 4

Foodborne disease outbreaks with known etiology by cause: United States, 1993–1997.

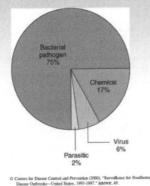

Bacterial pathogen 75%

Chemical 17%

Virus 6%

Parasitic 2%

© Centers for Disease Control and Prevention (2000). "Surveillance for Foodborne Disease Outbreaks—United States, 1993-1997." *MMWR*, 49.

© 2008 Jones and Bartlett Publishers, Inc. (www.jbpub.com)

Biological Hazards & Human Health - 4

- **Prevention of foodborne diseases**
  - Coordinated effort of federal, state, & local health agencies
  - Federal level: FoodNet– tracks 9 foodborne diseases in 8 catchment areas
  - Enforcement of state regulations at the local level is the job of sanitarians (registered environmental health specialists) through inspections
  - Consumers can reduce the risk of foodborne diseases by following safe food-handling recommendations

© 2008 Jones and Bartlett Publishers, Inc. (www.jbpub.com)

Biological Hazards & Human Health - 5

- **Vectorborne diseases:** diseases spread by a vector (a living organism, usually an insect or other arthropod, that transmits microscopic disease agents to susceptible host) e.g., of vectors– mosquitoes, fleas, lice, ticks
- **Vectorborne disease outbreak (VBDO):** the occurrence of 2 or more cases of a vectorborne disease; e.g., diseases– St. Louis encephalitis, West Nile virus
- **Prevention of VBDOs:** remove standing water (e.g., discarded car tires) that provide habitats in which vectors can proliferate, & use insect repellant

© 2008 Jones and Bartlett Publishers, Inc. (www.jbpub.com)

Notes

Biological Hazards & Human Health - 6

Table 16.2
Vectorborne Biological Hazards

Hazard	Agent	Vector	Disease
Virus	SLE virus	Mosquito	St. Louis encephalitis
	LaCrosse	Mosquito	LaCrosse encephalitis
Rickettsiae	Rickettsia typhi	Flea	Murine typhus
	Rickettsia rickettsii	Tick	Rocky Mountain spotted fever
	Ehrlichia chaffeensis	Tick	Ehrlichiosis
Bacteria	Yersinia pestis	Flea	Bubonic plague
	Borrelia burgdorferi	Tick	Lyme disease
Protozoa	Plasmodium spp.	Mosquito	Malaria
Nematodes	Wuchereria bancrofti	Mosquito	Filariasis (elephantiasis)

Source: Chin, J., ed. (2000). *Control of Communicable Diseases Manual*, 17th ed. Washington, DC: American Public Health Association.

© 2008 Jones and Bartlett Publishers, Inc. (www.jbpub.com)

Chemical Hazards & Human Health - 1

- **Chemical hazards**: those caused by the mismanagement of chemicals

- **Children are much more vulnerable to chemical assaults than adults**

- **Three common ones– pesticides, environmental tobacco smoke, & lead**

© 2008 Jones and Bartlett Publishers, Inc. (www.jbpub.com)

Chemical Hazards & Human Health - 2

- **Pest:** any organism (plant, animal, or microbe) that has an adverse effect on human interests

- **Pesticides:** natural or synthetic chemicals that have been developed & manufactured for the purpose of killing pests; 25,000 in the U.S.

- **Most widely used pesticides are herbicides (kill plants) & insecticides (kill insects)**

© 2008 Jones and Bartlett Publishers, Inc. (www.jbpub.com)

Chemical Hazards & Human Health - 3

- **Pesticide poisonings:** occur most frequently with children & workers who apply pesticides; consumed orally, inhaled, or when they come in contact with skin

- **Children:** most orally; most unintentional

- **Workers:** most often from careless practice; farm workers misuse of pesticides; e.g., illiterate & unable to read instructions

Chemical Hazards & Human Health - 4

- **Most pesticides are aimed at a single pest (target pest or target organism) but will kill many**
- **Ideal pesticide**
  - Inexpensive
  - Kills only target organism
  - Breaks down rapidly
  - Breaks down into harmless chemicals
- **Immediate solutions:** better education about safe storage & proper use, better regulations, & better compliance with instructions

Chemical Hazards & Human Health - 5

- **Environmental tobacco smoke (ETS) or secondhand smoke**
  - Class A carcinogen; 3,000 deaths per year; many other health-related effects
  - Smoke: sidestream smoke (off the end of a burning cigarette); mainstream smoke (smoker inhales & exhales)
  - Passive smoking: inhaling ETS; none risk-free
- Education on hazards of ETS
- Regulation necessitated by those who think smoking is a right
- Policy to provide smoke-free workplaces; best if voluntary

Notes

Chemical Hazards & Human Health - 6

- **Lead:** naturally occurring mineral element that is found throughout the environment & used in industrial products, e.g., pipe, paint, solder

- **Humans exposed by:** ingestion & inhalation; children at greatest risk via lead-based paint dust

- **Health concerns:** chronic in nature; can cause anemia, birth defects, bone damage, neurological damage, kidney damage

---

Chemical Hazards & Human Health - 7

- **Prevention of lead poisoning:** includes education, regulation, & prudent behavior
- **RCRA & the Comprehensive Environmental Response, Compensation, & Liability Act (CERCLA):** helped to regulate the disposal of lead-based products
- **The Lead Contamination Control Act of 1988:** has allowed the CDC to provide grants to allow states to do the following: screen infants & children for elevated lead levels, ensure referral for medical & environmental intervention, provide education to parents & children about lead poisoning

---

Physical Hazards & Human Health - 1

- **Physical hazards can impact human health:** e.g., temperature, equipment & environmental design, & radiation

- **Radiation:** release of energy when atoms are split or decay; energy can cause cells to mutate or die

- **Radon gas contamination:** radon gas comes from rocks & soil; harmless when it disperses into the air, but when trapped in a building can cause great harm; 2nd leading cause of lung cancer

---

Physical Hazards & Human Health - 2

- **Radon gas**
  - Enters buildings through the following: cracks in the foundation walls & floor, joints, openings around sump pump drains, loose-fitting pipes, & porous building materials
  - Consumed by inhaling through the air or water
  - All homes should be tested for radon; if found it can be fixed for anywhere between $800 & $2000

Physical Hazards & Human Health - 3

- **Ultraviolet (UV) radiation:** radiation energy with wavelengths 0-400 nanometers (nm)
- **UV-B (290-330 nm):** cause the most harm to humans; skin cancers; 1,000,000 new cases each year; most common skin cancers– basal & squamous cell
- **Prevention of & solutions to UV radiation exposure:** reduce exposure; seek early treatment
- **What to look for:** ABCDs = asymmetry, border irregularity, color, diameter

Psychological Hazards & Human Health

- **Psychological hazards effects are hard to quantify**

- **Health problems:** hypochondriasis, depression, hysteria, & stress

- **Concern today:** international terrorism; produce state of fear, stress, & hysteria

- **9/11:** much trauma; concern with post-traumatic stress disorder (PTSD)

Sociological Hazards & Human Health - 1

- **Living around others can create sociological hazards**

- **Noise, overcrowding, traffic jams, isolation, lack of privacy, & crowds influence human health– but exact impact unknown**

- **Population growth:** influenced by birth rate, death rate, & migration– but with world population migration is not a factor; explained by S & J-curves

© 2008 Jones and Bartlett Publishers, Inc. (www.jbpub.com)

Sociological Hazards & Human Health - 2

World Population Growth

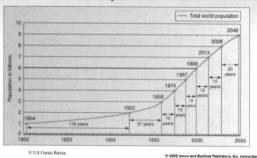

© U.S Census Bureau

© 2008 Jones and Bartlett Publishers, Inc. (www.jbpub.com)

Sociological Hazards & Human Health - 3

- **Carrying capacity:** maximum population size that can be supported by available resources (air, water, shelter, etc.)
- **The facts–**
  - World's 6 billionth person was born in 1999; growth rate will decline but size will grow; 9.4 billion by 2050
  - 80% of world's population lives in less developed countries; greatest expected growth to be in sub-Saharan Africa
  - U.S. growth will continue mostly because of migration

© 2008 Jones and Bartlett Publishers, Inc. (www.jbpub.com)

Sociological Hazards & Human Health - 4

- **Population growth issues**
  - Can quality of life be continued with growth?
  - Environmental issues: global warming, acid rain, depletion of the ozone, increasing crime rates, increasing vulnerability to epidemics & pandemics, smog, contamination of soils & groundwater, degradation of land, & international tensions
  - Urban areas continue to grow: number of megacities (>10 million people): 5 in 1975, 19 now, & 23 expected by 2015

© 2008 Jones and Bartlett Publishers, Inc. (www.jbpub.com)

Sociological Hazards & Human Health - 5

- **Population growth solutions**
  - Most experts feel the world population is reaching maximum sustainable limit, though no one knows what the carrying capacity is
  - Growth rate slowed to 1.2%
  - Human means of dealing with the issues: (1) various methods of conception control, (2) birth control methods, & (3) social policies dealing with financial incentives & disincentives
  - Alternative is to let nature take its course (famine, epidemics, & perhaps warfare)

© 2008 Jones and Bartlett Publishers, Inc. (www.jbpub.com)

Natural Disasters & Human Health - 1

- **Natural disasters:** those geophysical & meteorological events (disaster agents) that greatly exceed normal human expectations in terms of magnitude or frequency & cause significant injury to individuals & damage to property
- **Primary needs after a disaster:** food, water, shelter, health care, clothing
- **Federal Emergency Response Agency (FEMA):** agency within the DHS; prepares communities for all hazards & manages the federal response & recovery efforts after any national incident
- **ARC:** provides relief to victims of disasters

© 2008 Jones and Bartlett Publishers, Inc. (www.jbpub.com)

Notes

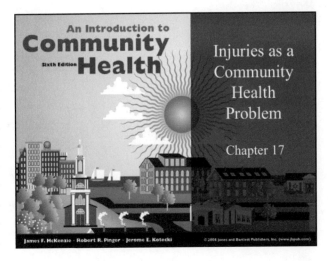

Key Definitions

- **Injury:** physical damage to the body resulting from mechanical, chemical, thermal, or other environmental energy

- **Unintentional injuries:** those that have occurred without anyone intending harm to be done

- **Intentional injuries:** those that have been purposely inflicted, either by the victim or another

© 2008 Jones and Bartlett Publishers, Inc. (www.jbpub.com)

Other Key Definitions

- **Accident:** the term has fallen into disfavor because it suggests a chance occurrence or unpreventable mishap; replaced with **unintentional injury**

- **Safety:** the term safety has been replaced by **injury prevention** or **injury control**

© 2008 Jones and Bartlett Publishers, Inc. (www.jbpub.com)

Characteristics of Unintentional Injuries

1. **Unplanned events**

2. **Preceded by an unsafe act (behavior) or condition (environmental factor)** [Note: unsafe acts or conditions are called hazards]

3. **Often accompanied by economic loss**

4. **Interrupt the efficient completion of tasks**

© 2008 Jones and Bartlett Publishers, Inc. (www.jbpub.com)

Cost of Injuries to Society

- **5.2 million deaths/year worldwide**
- **150,000+ deaths/year in the U. S.;** 5th leading cause; 3rd in YPLL for unintentional; 1st for combined unintentional & intentional
- **~11% of world's disease burden is caused by injuries**
- **156 million medically attended injury-related episodes/yr. in U. S.**
- **$575 billion/year on unintentional injuries**
- **Great burden on emergency departments**

© 2008 Jones and Bartlett Publishers, Inc. (www.jbpub.com)

Cost of Injuries to Society

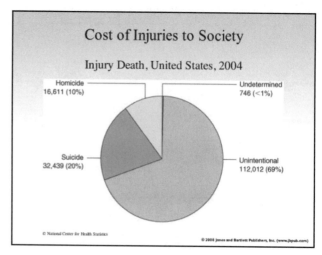

Injury Death, United States, 2004

Homicide 16,611 (10%)
Undetermined 746 (<1%)
Suicide 32,439 (20%)
Unintentional 112,012 (69%)

© National Center for Health Statistics

© 2008 Jones and Bartlett Publishers, Inc. (www.jbpub.com)

Cost of Injuries to Society

Burden of Injury, United States, 2004

Deaths
161,808

Disabling injuries
23,200,000

Emergency department visits
41,400,000

Medically attended injuries
156,000,000

©National Center for Health Statistics and the National Safety Council

© 2008 Jones and Bartlett Publishers, Inc. (www.jbpub.com)

Unintentional Injuries - 1

- **In 2004, 112,012 unintentional injury deaths in U.S.**

- **Major causes:** motor vehicle crashes (40%); poisonings (18%); & falls (17%)

- **Cost: $575 billion:** $298 billion from lost wages; $99 billion in medical expenses; $112 billion insurance administration; $65 billion from vehicle damage & other

© 2008 Jones and Bartlett Publishers, Inc. (www.jbpub.com)

Unintentional Injuries - 2

- **Motor vehicle crashes**
  - #1 cause of unintentional injury deaths in the World & U.S.; only 10% of the deaths in developed countries
  - In U.S. in 2005, 2 million crashes, 1.9 million injuries, & 43,433 fatalities
  - Most deaths were to drivers (64%), then passengers (28%), motorcycle drivers (3%), pedestrians (3%), and pedacyclists (2%)
  - Injury rates per vehicle miles traveled has dropped slightly

© 2008 Jones and Bartlett Publishers, Inc. (www.jbpub.com)

Unintentional Injuries - 3

- **Poisonings**
  - #2 cause of unintentional injury deaths in the U.S.; 19,250 deaths; result from ingestion of medicines & drugs, toxic foods (e.g., mushrooms & shellfish), & occupational materials; 80% occur in the home
- **Falls**
  - #3 cause of unintentional injury deaths in the U.S.; 18,535 deaths; leading cause of ED visits; most occur in homes; disproportionately affect elders
- **Other deaths from:** fires & burns (3,223), drownings (3,180), other transport (2,986), & firearms (661)

© 2008 Jones and Bartlett Publishers, Inc. (www.jbpub.com)

Epidemiology of Unintentional Injuries - 1

- **Person (Who?)**
  - Age: leading cause of death in the 1 to 44-years age group, most (by motor vehicles); children & teenagers (firearms); elders (falls)
  - Gender: males twice as likely to be affected than females
  - Minority status: leading cause of death for 1 to 34 years for all racial and ethnic groups except blacks; highest for American Indian/Alaskan Natives; lowest for Asian/Pacific Islanders

© 2008 Jones and Bartlett Publishers, Inc. (www.jbpub.com)

Epidemiology of Unintentional Injuries - 2

- **Place (Where?)**
  - Home: more unintentional injuries occur in the home than in any other place
  - Highways: rank 2nd for nonfatal injuries; ranks 1st for unintentional injury deaths
  - Recreation/sports area: 3rd mostly likely place to sustain injury
  - Workplace: 4th highest rate of unintentional injuries; mining, farming (includes logging), & construction

© 2008 Jones and Bartlett Publishers, Inc. (www.jbpub.com)

Notes

Epidemiology of Unintentional Injuries - 3

Number and Percentage of Where Injuries Occur

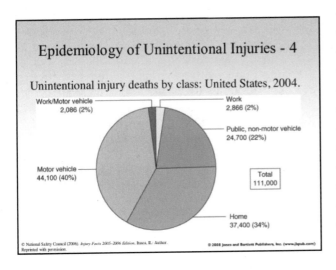

- Street/Highway/Parking lot 4,449 (13.4%)
- Sport facility/Recreation area/Lake/River 4,003 (12.1%)
- Workplace 3,080 (9.3%)
- School/Child care center/Preschool 2,598 (7.8%)
- Other 2,151 (6.5%)
- Hospital/Residential institution 554 (1.7%)
- Home 15,268 (46.3%)

© Data from Adams, P. F., et al. (2006). *Vital and Health Statistics,* 10(229): 1–104.   © 2008 Jones and Bartlett Publishers, Inc. (www.jbpub.com)

Epidemiology of Unintentional Injuries - 4

Unintentional injury deaths by class: United States, 2004.

- Work/Motor vehicle 2,086 (2%)
- Work 2,866 (2%)
- Public, non-motor vehicle 24,700 (22%)
- Motor vehicle 44,100 (40%)
- Home 37,400 (34%)
- Total 111,000

© National Safety Council (2006). *Injury Facts 2005–2006 Edition.* Itasca, IL: Author. Reprinted with permission.   © 2008 Jones and Bartlett Publishers, Inc. (www.jbpub.com)

Epidemiology of Unintentional Injuries - 5

- **Time (When?)**
  - Deaths from unintentional injuries have fallen over past 30+ years
  - Seasonal variations
  - Motor vehicle crashes: highest rate in November & December; more deaths occur on Fridays through Sundays; alcohol is involved in 40% of fatal crashes
  - Drowning: more occur in the summer months; alcohol is involved in nearly 1/2
  - Fires: more occur November to April

© 2008 Jones and Bartlett Publishers, Inc. (www.jbpub.com)

Notes

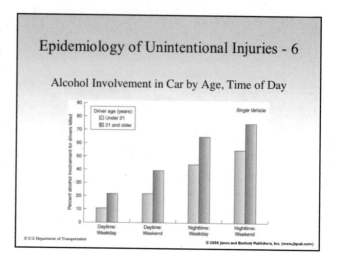

Epidemiology of Unintentional Injuries - 6

Alcohol Involvement in Car by Age, Time of Day

Prevention through Epidemiology - 1

- **Most implementation of prevention activities related to injuries occurs only after costly disasters**
- **First important efforts toward injury prevention & control began early in 20th century**
- **Injury Prevention & Control Contributors:** Hugh De Haven (studied falls), John E. Gordon (used epidemiology), James Gibson (energy transfer), William Haddon, Jr. (lack of energy; father of injury prevention research)

© 2008 Jones and Bartlett Publishers, Inc. (www.jbpub.com)

Prevention through Epidemiology - 2

- **Little progress to reducing unintentional injuries & deaths until the 1950s;** in part because no causative agent identified

- **Model for unintentional injuries:** similar to communicable disease model except the agent is "energy" in this model

- **Transfer of energy**

© 2008 Jones and Bartlett Publishers, Inc. (www.jbpub.com)

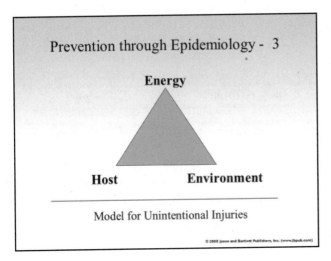

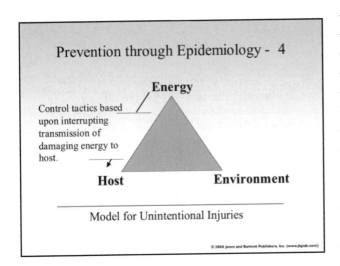

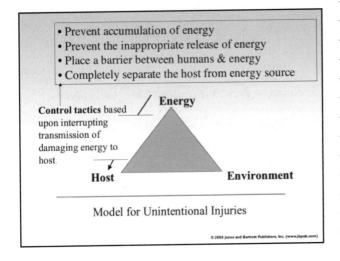

Notes

Community Approach to Prevention of Unintentional Injuries - 1

- **Education:** injury prevention education– the process of changing people's health-directed behavior so as to reduce unintentional injuries

- **Regulation:** the enactment & enforcement of laws to control conduct; e.g., 55 MPH, child safety seats, BAC 0.08%; need to consider a "free society"

© 2008 Jones and Bartlett Publishers, Inc. (www.jbpub.com)

Community Approach to Prevention of Unintentional Injuries - 2

- **Automatic (or passive) protection:** the modification of a product or environment so as to reduce unintentional injuries; e.g., child-proof safety caps, air bags in motor vehicles

- **Litigation:** the process of seeking justice for injury through courts; e.g., removing dangerous products from the shelves

© 2008 Jones and Bartlett Publishers, Inc. (www.jbpub.com)

Intentional Injuries

- **Intentional injuries:** the result of self-directed or interpersonal violence; ~50,000 people die each year; millions more are injured; highest rates in males & females 20-24 years old & in black males
- **Types:** range from assaults, rape, robberies, suicides, homicides, family violence (children, elders, partners); suicides, 11th leading cause of death; homicides & legal intervention, 13th leading cause
- **Problem for communities:** loss of life, productivity, money, and consume many community resources

© 2008 Jones and Bartlett Publishers, Inc. (www.jbpub.com)

Notes

Epidemiology of Intentional Injuries - 1

- **Disproportionately affect those who are frustrated, hopeless, jobless, live in poverty, & those with low self-esteem**

- **More acts committed by males & those who have been abused or neglected**

- **Alcohol & drugs often involved; firearms are increasingly involved**

© 2008 Jones and Bartlett Publishers, Inc. (www.jbpub.com)

Epidemiology of Intentional Injuries - 2

- **Homicide, assault, and rape:** homicide rate 5.5 per 100,000; declining rates in last 15 yrs.; risk factors (< 25 years old, poor, males, black); handguns a problem
- **Suicide & attempted suicide**: nearly 30,000 suicides are reported each year; rates among the young people have tripled since 1950; higher in males
- **Firearm injuries & injury deaths:** 2nd leading cause of injury death; 67% of homicide & 54% of suicides involved a firearm; highest risk young males; no detailed federal supported reporting system

© 2008 Jones and Bartlett Publishers, Inc. (www.jbpub.com)

Epidemiology of Intentional Injuries - 3

Firearm Injury Versus Other Types of Injury

© Centers for Disease Control and Prevention

© 2008 Jones and Bartlett Publishers, Inc. (www.jbpub.com)

Violence in Our Society & Resources for Prevention - 1

- **Overview:** violence in America has increased in past few years; many lack skills for conflict resolution; firearms make violence more deadly

- **Individuals & violence:** lack communication & problem-solving skills; not interested in resolving but rather "winning"; firearms are easy to obtain & deadly; homicide & legal intervention #1 cause of death in black Americans aged 15-24 years; more violence prevention programs in schools

© 2008 Jones and Bartlett Publishers, Inc. (www.jbpub.com)

Violence in Our Society & Resources for Prevention - 2

- **Family violence & abuse**
  - Family violence: the use of physical force by one family member against another, with the intent to hurt, injure, or cause death

  - 1 in 6 homicides is the result of family violence

  - Need to intervene in family violence

© 2008 Jones and Bartlett Publishers, Inc. (www.jbpub.com)

Violence in Our Society & Resources for Prevention - 3

Decline in Child Maltreatment Rates

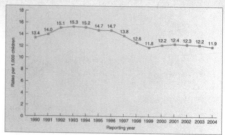

© Department of Health and Human Services

© 2008 Jones and Bartlett Publishers, Inc. (www.jbpub.com)

Violence in Our Society & Resources for Prevention - 4

Child Maltreatment According to Age of the Child

© Department of Health and Human Services

© 2008 Jones and Bartlett Publishers, Inc. (www.jbpub.com)

Violence in Our Society & Resources for Prevention - 5

- **Family violence & abuse (continued)**
  - Child maltreatment: an act or failure to act that results in physical abuse, neglect, medical neglect, sexual abuse, emotional abuse, or presents an imminent risk of serious harm
  - Child abuse: can be physical, emotional, verbal, or sexual
  - Child neglect: maltreatment
  - Prevention: need for timely reporting & referral; Child Protection Service (CPS) agencies

© 2008 Jones and Bartlett Publishers, Inc. (www.jbpub.com)

Violence in Our Society & Resources for Prevention - 6

- **Family violence & abuse (continued)**
  - Elder maltreatment: rates lower than other age groups; includes abuse, neglect, exploitation, & mistreatment; women over 75 years most vulnerable; 90% of abusers are family members
  - Intimate partner violence (IPV): rates declining, but still too high; risk factors (poor, living with those who abuse alcohol & drugs); cycle of violence; prevention; identifying & documenting cases & increased access to services

© 2008 Jones and Bartlett Publishers, Inc. (www.jbpub.com)

Notes

Violence in Our Society &
Resources for Prevention - 7

Power and Abusive Partners

© Data from AHEC News (February, 1996), 2(1): 9. Used with permission.
© 2008 Jones and Bartlett Publishers, Inc. (www.jbpub.com)

Violence in Our Society &
Resources for Prevention - 8

- **Violence in Schools**
  - Schools are one of the safest places, but there is still violence
  - Several high-profile situations: Columbine H.S., Virginia Tech University; Amish school in PA
  - ~3/4 of schools have reported one or more violent acts in a year; many with weapons
  - Zero tolerance policies
  - Bullying & being bullied an increasing problem

© 2008 Jones and Bartlett Publishers, Inc. (www.jbpub.com)

Violence in Our Society &
Resources for Prevention - 9

- **Violence in Schools (continued)**
  - *Safe Schools/Healthy Student Initiatives*: grant program from U.S. Departments of Education, HHS, & Justice; 7-step process; requires comprehensive, integrated community-wide plans
  - Youth violence after school; lack of adult supervision after school & youth are more vulnerable to exploitation, injuries & even death
  - Communities can use *Best Practices of Youth Violence Prevention: A Sourcebook for Community Action*

© 2008 Jones and Bartlett Publishers, Inc. (www.jbpub.com)

Violence in Our Society & Resources for Prevention - 10

- **Violence in Communities**
  - Youth gang: a self-formed association of peers bound together by mutual interests, with identifiable leadership & well-defined lines of authority; organized subculture; found in 29% of U.S.; prevalent in cities with > 25,000 people

  - Cost to communities: youth gangs are a great drain on community resources; vandalism & graffiti real problems

© 2008 Jones and Bartlett Publishers, Inc. (www.jbpub.com)

Violence in Our Society & Resources for Prevention - 11

- **Violence in Communities (continued)**
  - Community response: multifaceted effort of law enforcement, education, diversion activities, & social support services

  - Federal government's response: Brady Handgun Violence Prevention Act (interstate trafficking of guns & waiting period); National Child Protection Act of 1993 (fingerprint-based national background check on individuals seeking employment in the child care field)

© 2008 Jones and Bartlett Publishers, Inc. (www.jbpub.com)

Chapter 18: Safety and Health in the Workplace

Notes

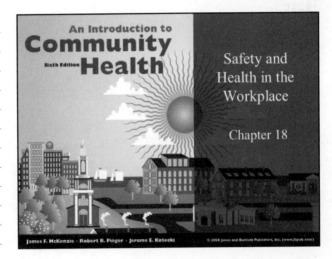

Introduction - 1

- **Worldwide**
  - 2.6 billion workers
  - Each year, 270 million occupational injuries, resulting in 351,000 fatalities
  - Each year, 160 million new cases of work-related diseases
- **United States**
  - 149+ million workers
  - Next to home, where Americans spend most of their time at work

© 2008 Jones and Bartlett Publishers, Inc. (www.jbpub.com)

Introduction - 2

- **Occupational disease:** an abnormal condition or disorder, other than one resulting from an occupational injury, caused by factors associated with employment

- **Occupational injury:** injury that results from exposure to a single incident in the work environment

© 2008 Jones and Bartlett Publishers, Inc. (www.jbpub.com)

Notes

History of Occupational Safety & Health Problems - 2

- **Occupational Safety & Health in the U.S. before 1970**
  - Industrial Revolution: 18th century in Britain, Europe then U.S.; movement from people power to machines
  - Unsafe occupations: mining, iron smelting, & cotton mills & textile factories
  - Injuries a concern before diseases

© 2008 Jones and Bartlett Publishers, Inc. (www.jbpub.com)

History of Occupational Safety & Health Problems - 3

- **Occupational Safety & Health in the U.S. before 1970 (continued)**
  - State legislation: in 1835 MA passed child labor law; in 1877 MA passed first worker safety law; 1902 MD became first state to pass workers' compensation law; 1948 MS became last state to pass workers' compensation law
  - Alice Hamilton (1869-1970): pioneer in occupational safety & health in U.S.; led crusades to reduce poisonings

© 2008 Jones and Bartlett Publishers, Inc. (www.jbpub.com)

History of Occupational Safety & Health Problems - 4

- **Occupational Safety & Health in the U.S. before 1970 (continued)**
  - Federal legislation: 1884 Bureau of Labor created; 1910 Federal Bureau of Mines; 1914 Office of Industrial Hygiene & Sanitation in the PHS
  - Many laws passed between 1908 & 1970
  - Most important: Occupational Safety and Health Act of 1970 (OSHAct)

© 2008 Jones and Bartlett Publishers, Inc. (www.jbpub.com)

Notes

Highlights of Federal Occupational Safety & Health Legislation - 1

Year	Legislation
1908	Federal Workmen's Compensation Act (limited coverage)
1916	Federal Highway Aid Act
1926	Federal Workmen's Compensation Act (included workers)
1927	Federal Longshoremen's & Harbor Workers' Compensation Act
1936	Walsh-Healey Public Contracts Act
1952	Coal Mine Safety Act
1959	Radiation Standards Act

© 2008 Jones and Bartlett Publishers, Inc. (www.jbpub.com)

Highlights of Federal Occupational Safety & Health Legislation - 2

Year	Legislation
1960	Federal Hazardous Substances Labeling Act
1966	National Traffic & Motor Vehicle Safety Act Child Protection Act (banned hazardous household substances)
1967	National Commission on Product Safety created
1968	Natural Gas Pipeline Safety Act
1969	Construction Safety Act Coal Mine Health & Safety Act
1970	Occupational Safety & Health Act

© 2008 Jones and Bartlett Publishers, Inc. (www.jbpub.com)

History of Occupational Safety & Health Problems - 5

- **Occupational Safety & Health Act of 1970**
  - Purpose: to ensure that employers in the private sector provide employees with a working environment free of recognized hazards that can cause death or serious harm
  - Formed Occupational Safety & Health Administration (OHSA): to create & enforce occupational standards
  - Formed National Institute for Occupational Safety & Health (NIOSH): research body now in CDC; recommends standards

© 2008 Jones and Bartlett Publishers, Inc. (www.jbpub.com)

Prevalence of Occupational Injuries, Disease, & Deaths

- **Overview of recent trends**
  - Since 1992, the numbers of injuries & illnesses have declined
  - In 2005 in U.S., 4.2 million injuries & diseases; 90% are injuries
  - In 2005, highest rates were in manufacturing (6.3/100 full-time workers), construction (6.3), & agriculture, forestry, & fishing (6.1)
  - Lowest rates: in finance, insurance, & real estate

© 2008 Jones and Bartlett Publishers, Inc. (www.jbpub.com)

Prevalence of Occupational Injuries, Disease, & Deaths

Nonfatal workplace injury and illness incidence rates by industry division, 2005.

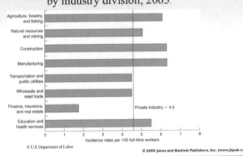

© U.S Department of Labor

© 2008 Jones and Bartlett Publishers, Inc. (www.jbpub.com)

Unintentional Injuries in the Workplace - 1

- **Unintentional injuries include both minor injuries (e.g., bruises, cuts) & major injuries (e.g., amputations, fractures)**
- **Fatal work-related injuries:** 16/day in U.S.; almost 6,000/year; highest rates per 100,000 are agriculture, forestry, fishing, hunting (32.5) & mining (25.6)
- **Nonfatal work-related injuries:** In 2003, 3.5 million occupational injuries & illnesses were treated in ERs; most common sprains & strains (24%) & lacerations, punctures, amputations, & avulsions (24%)
- **Disabling injuries:** those that keep worker away from job beyond the day he/she was injured

© 2008 Jones and Bartlett Publishers, Inc. (www.jbpub.com)

Notes

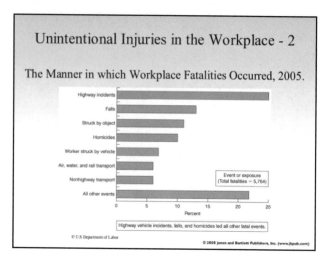

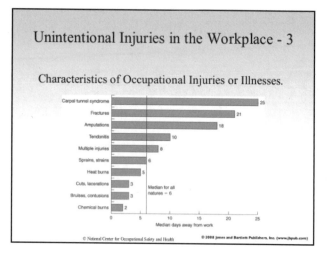

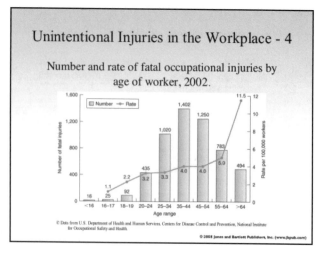

Unintentional Injuries in the Workplace - 5

- **Characteristics of injured workers**
  - Age: injuries lowest for 16-19 year olds; death rates highest for 65+ age group; youth who work > 20 hours per wk. do worse academically & are more likely to abuse drugs & alcohol; a concern is violation of child labor laws
  - Gender: almost 1/2 of workers are women; over 1/2 of women work; men work more hours and ~2/3 of all injury & illness involving days away from work involve men; women who work are more likely to have health benefits (e.g., insurance, health education) than nonworking women

Unintentional Injuries in the Workplace - 6

- **Characteristics of injured workers**
  - Poverty & race: nonwhites have highest death rates; Asians have the lowest death rates; other death rates vary depending on type of work performed
  - Geographic differences: Alaska & Wyoming are the states with the highest occupational death rates; rates higher in rural areas
  - Temporal variations: 81% decline in deaths from injuries between 1912 & 2005; death rates vary on season of the year & type of work

Unintentional Injuries in the Workplace - 7

Number & Rate of Fatal Occupational Injuries by Private Industry Sector, 2005.

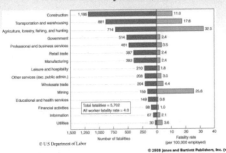

Unintentional Injuries in the Workplace - 8

Table 18.2
Top Ten Most Dangerous Jobs in 2005

Rank	Occupation	Death Rate/ 100,000	Total Deaths
1	Fishers and fishing workers	118.4	48
2	Logging workers	92.9	80
3	Aircraft pilots	66.9	81
4	Structural iron and steel workers	55.6	35
5	Refuse and recyclable material collectors	43.8	32
6	Farmers and ranchers	41.1	341
7	Electrical power line installers/repairers	32.7	36
8	Driver/sales workers and truck drivers	29.1	993
9	Miscellaneous agricultural workers	23.2	176
10	Construction laborers	22.7	339

© 2008 Jones and Bartlett Publishers, Inc. (www.jbpub.com)

Workplace Injuries by Industry & Occupation - 1

- **Nonfatal occupational injuries & illness by industry**
  - Goods-producing sector: highest injury rate in manufacturing

  - Service-producing sector: highest rate in transportation & warehousing

© 2008 Jones and Bartlett Publishers, Inc. (www.jbpub.com)

Workplace Injuries by Industry & Occupation - 2

- **Agriculture Safety & Health**
  - Farmers are at considerable risk for injuries, lung diseases, noise-induced hearing loss, skin diseases, & certain cancers
  - Farm machinery associated with many deaths, especially the tractor; tractor rollovers a concern: since 1985 tractors include seat belts & rollover protective structures (ROPS)
  - Concern for youth farm workers
  - Migrant at great risk for injury & diseases

© 2008 Jones and Bartlett Publishers, Inc. (www.jbpub.com)

Prevention & Control of Unintentional Injuries in the Workplace

- **Reduction of injuries involves 4 fundamental tasks**:
  - Anticipation: of future adverse events & to prevent them
  - Recognition: surveillance & monitoring of injuries & diseases
  - Evaluation: assessment of data
  - Control: interventions to improve safety
- **Leadership comes from OHSA & NIOSH**

© 2008 Jones and Bartlett Publishers, Inc. (www.jbpub.com)

Workplace Violence - 1

- **1.7 million Americans are victims of workplace violence each year**
- **Categories of workplace violence:** Criminal intent (Type I), Customer/client (Type II), Worker-on-worker (Type III), Personal relationship (Type IV)
- **Most assaults occur in service settings such as:** hospitals, nursing homes, & social service agencies
- **Risk factors:** contact with public; exchange of money; delivery; mobile workplace; working alone, at night, in high-crime areas, with unstable people; while guarding something; working in a community setting

© 2008 Jones and Bartlett Publishers, Inc. (www.jbpub.com)

Workplace Violence - 2

- **Prevention strategies**
  - First a workplace violence prevention policy should be in place
  - Environmental design: safe cash-handling procedures; separate workers from customers; better lighting; security system at entrances & exits
  - Administrative controls: staffing policies; procedures for opening & closing; reviewing employee duties that are risky
  - Behavior strategies: training employees in nonviolent response, conflict resolution, & risks associated with work

© 2008 Jones and Bartlett Publishers, Inc. (www.jbpub.com)

Notes

Occupational Illnesses & Disorders - 1

- **More difficult to get data on occupational illnesses than injuries**
- **Data show that illnesses account for ~6% of occupational injury & illness cases**
- **Types of occupational illnesses**
  - Musculoskeletal conditions: most frequent type; repeated trauma disorder 65% of all cases
  - Skin disease & disorders: number of cases have dropped by 50% in last 20 years; allergic & irritant dermatitis most common

Occupational Illnesses & Disorders - 2

- **Types of occupational illnesses (continued)**
  - Noise-induced hearing loss another form of repeated trauma; most in manufacturing
  - Respiratory disorders: result from inhalation of toxic substances; most common work-related asthma (WRA); concerns– pneumoconiosis, asbestosis, silicosis, & byssinosis; chronic in nature
  - Other work-related diseases & disorders: poisoning & infections; infectious disease agents; antineoplastic drug exposure; anxiety, stress, or neurotic disorders

Prevention & Control of Occupational Diseases & Disorders

- **Agent-host-environment model**
  - Identification & evaluation of agents; standard setting for handling & exposure to causative agents; elimination/substitution of causative factors
  - Medical screenings & care, & health promotion
  - Engineering controls to provide safe areas
  - Protective devices
  - Disease surveillance & environmental monitoring

Agent

Environment   Host

Notes

Resources for Prevention of Workplace Injuries & Diseases - 1

- **Safety & health professionals**
  - Safety engineers & certified safety professionals (CSP): design safety education programs, & detect hazards & correct them
  - Health physicists: concerned with radiation in the workplace
  - Industrial hygienists: concerned with environmental factors that might cause illness

© 2008 Jones and Bartlett Publishers, Inc. (www.jbpub.com)

Resources for Prevention of Workplace Injuries & Diseases - 2

- **Safety & health professionals (continued)**
  - Occupational physicians (OP) or occupational medical practitioner (OMP): occupational medicine; concerned with preventive medicine in the workplace
  - Occupational health nurse (OHN): moved from running first-aid station to health promotion & illness prevention

© 2008 Jones and Bartlett Publishers, Inc. (www.jbpub.com)

Resources for Prevention of Workplace Injuries & Diseases - 3

- **Occupational Safety & Health Programs**
  - There are a number of programs that can be put in place to reduce workplace injuries & illness
  - Pre-placement examinations: to make sure that the employee is mentally & physically fit for the job
  - Occupational disease prevention & safety programs: aimed at reducing disease because of exposure & injury by policies, procedures, & plans for prevention

© 2008 Jones and Bartlett Publishers, Inc. (www.jbpub.com)

Notes

Resources for Prevention of Workplace
Injuries & Diseases - 4

- **Occupational Safety & Health Programs
  (continued)**
  - Worksite health promotion (WHP) programs: are
    workplace-based programs aimed at improving the
    health of employees through changes in behavior &
    lifestyle; used to help reduce the health care bill of
    insured employees
  - Employee assistance programs (EAPs): those that
    help employees who have substance abuse, domestic,
    psychological, or social problems that interfere with
    work performance

© 2008 Jones and Bartlett Publishers, Inc. (www.jbpub.com)